Equine Behaviour: Principles and Practice

D.S. Mills

and

K.J. Nankervis

Blackwell
Science

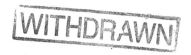

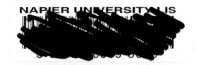

© 1999 by Blackwell Science Ltd,
a Blackwell Publishing Company
Editorial Offices:
9600 Garsington Rd, Oxford, OX4 2DQ
 Tel: +44 (0)1865 206206
Blackwell Science, Inc., 350 Main Street,
Malden, MA 02148-5018, USA
 Tel: +1 781 388 8250
Iowa State Press, a Blackwell Publishing
Company, 2121 State Avenue, Ames, Iowa
50014-8300, USA
 Tel: +1 515 292 0140
Blackwell Science Asia Pty, 54 University
Street, Carlton, Victoria 3053, Australia
 Tel: +61 (0)3 9347 0300
Blackwell Wissenschafts Verlag,
Kurfürstendamm 57, 10707 Berlin, Germany
 Tel: +49 (0)30 32 79 060

First published 1999 by Blackwell Science Ltd
Reprinted 2001, 2002, 2003

Library of Congress
Cataloging-in-Publication Data
Mills, D.S.
    Equine behaviour: principles and
 practice/D.S. Mills and K.J. Nankervis.
        p.   cm.
    Includes bibliographical references and
 index.
    ISBN 0-632-04878-6 (pbk.)
    1. Horses – Behavior.   I. Nankervis, K.J.
 II. Title.
 SF281.M58   1999
 636.1 – dc21   98-55558
                                           CIP

ISBN 0-632-04878-6

A catalogue record for this title is available
from the British Library

Set in 10.5/12.5pt Palatino
by DP Photosetting, Aylesbury, Bucks
Printed and bound in Great Britain by
MPG Books Ltd, Bodmin, Cornwall

For further information on
Blackwell Publishing, visit our website:
www.blackwellpublishing.com

Contents

Preface

Almost everyone who feels qualified to call himself or herself a horse-person will have studied equine behaviour to a certain extent. Initial interest in equine behaviour often arises when we have a problem and ask 'Why won't my horse do what I want it to do?' Thereafter, naturally, the study of equine behaviour is motivated from a 'How can I get it to do what I want?' standpoint. It is very easy, then, to look for 'recipes' which sort out the current problem but which fail to address the underlying, often fundamental issue.

The answer to our first question may simply be 'because it is a horse'. If only we were to understand what being a horse is about, then we would recognise that the problem lies with us, either in our approach to a situation, or in our expectations of the horse. We must learn to accept that, however knowledgeable we are in the business of training horses, we cannot get around the fact that our two species have fundamental differences in priorities. If we insist then, on riding on and competing with horses, we should strive to do it to the best of our ability, so that both parties come out feeling like winners. Xenophon summed it up bluntly two and a half thousand years ago when he wrote:

> 'Seeing that you are forced to meddle with horses, don't you think that common sense requires you to see that you are not ignorant of the business?'

It is hoped that this book will go some way towards addressing this need, in a perhaps light-hearted fashion that nevertheless should not belie the basic seriousness of the concern we should all feel for the welfare of the horses in our care.

D.S. Mills
De Montfort University

K.J. Nankervis
Newmarket

August 1998

Acknowledgements

This book is based on lectures given by us to De Montfort University students over the last few years. It therefore owes a lot to them for their comments on what were, in effect, practice drafts of the original text. We are also grateful to Christine Nicol, Debbie Goodwin and Jonathan Cooper for comments on an earlier draft of the text. We would also like to thank our publishers for their support (and patience) during the book's production, and Tamsin Bacchus for her work in copy editing the text. Finally, we would also like to thank our partners, Connie and Tom, for all their help throughout.

This book is dedicated to everyone who has a serious interest in improving the welfare of horses, through a better understanding of their behaviour.

Part 1
Understanding Behaviour Concepts

In this section we introduce the principles behind the study and interpretation of animal behaviour. Anyone can watch animal behaviour but that is not the same as making a scientific study of it. In order to do this, we must understand and apply certain rules. An explanation of these helps us to understand why a horse behaves in a certain way, as well as why it does not behave in another way (the limits of its behaviour). These limitations are just as important when we consider how we should manage our horse best. With such understanding we are also in a position to test our own ideas scientifically with either field or laboratory experiments. This is the way in which scientific knowledge increases and our understanding of the needs of the horse improves.

1. *Approaches to the Study of Behaviour*

We may be motivated in our study of behaviour by the hope that we can improve the performance of our own horse in some particular way, seeking to make it do what we want, but in studying horse behaviour and its origins and management in general terms, we should not forget that not all horses are winners. You may be disappointed that the horse you had high hopes for turns out to be completely talentless, despite your strenuous efforts to 'understand' him. The problem may not lie with the method used, but with the potential of the horse. In other words, the horse's behaviour is a product of both its biology and its environment or 'nature and nurture', as many people call it. We should not get so wrapped up in our role in 'nurturing', that we forget about the 'nature' of horses in general and that horse in particular.

What is behaviour?

Behaviour is what living animals do, and what dead animals don't do. Behaviour is an expression of physiology. There are two broad ways in which we tend to describe behaviour:

(1) We can detail the physical actions involved in a behaviour; how one part moves relative to either another part of the body or the environment. For example, we might say that a horse has extended its foreleg, or that it is galloping.

(2) Alternatively we may describe the consequences of the behaviour or the suspected aim. For example, we might say that one horse is threatening or attacking another. This will often involve an element of interpretation, which can cause problems.

A horse dozing in a field is performing just as much behaviour as a horse that is fighting, riding a bike, or turning somersaults! These are all complex actions which involve the integration of several behavioural acts. The mechanism that allows a horse to sleep standing up is, in itself, a really neat piece of engineering. Contrary to popular belief, however, horses still need to spend a certain amount of time lying down in order to sleep properly. Management can have an effect on even this. Houpt (1991) reports that horses which are usually stabled sleep less for the first month after turn out, and do not even get down to sleep on the first night. Since sleep is essential for the normal functioning of an animal during its waking hours we should not be surprised if the performance of the horse is affected by such a management change. This simple example highlights an important theme: we cannot understand an animal's behaviour without referring to its environment. Horses do certain things in certain environments.

Why do horses gallop?

Niko Tinbergen pointed out that if we wanted to know why an animal performs a certain behaviour, there are always four very different, but equally correct answers. For example, if we ask the question, 'why do horses gallop?' the answer could be:

◇ 'Because nerve impulses from the brain and spinal cord lead to muscle contraction in a co-ordinated way to bring about the galloping gait'.

We could go even further by saying that the nerve impulses and muscle contractions occurred because of certain physiological and biochemical changes, and give a string of chemical equations in order to explain why the horse was galloping. This is the most basic answer, looking at the horse as though it were a piece of machinery. This answer, where the idea is to try and explain the behaviour in terms of its immediate cause and control, explains the causation of behaviour.

◇ 'Because during its early development the foal learned how to co-ordinate its limbs and body to allow it to gallop'.

This approach is to explain the behaviour in terms of the developmental history (the ontogeny) of the behaviour within an individual.

◇ 'Because, over millions of years, those ancient relatives of the horse which did not move so quickly and efficiently lost out and left no descendants. Horses gallop because that is how they have evolved to move most efficiently at high speed.'

This explains the behaviour in terms of its development not within an animal's lifetime history but within the history of the species. The evolutionary history of a behaviour explains how it is adapted to its environment and is often referred to as its phylogeny.

◇ Because galloping is the best way for a horse to avoid a predator.'

This offers an explanation as to the function of the behaviour. The function of the behaviour tells us its survival value.

The first two answers explain how a horse manages to gallop, whilst answers three and four consider the purpose of galloping,

causation

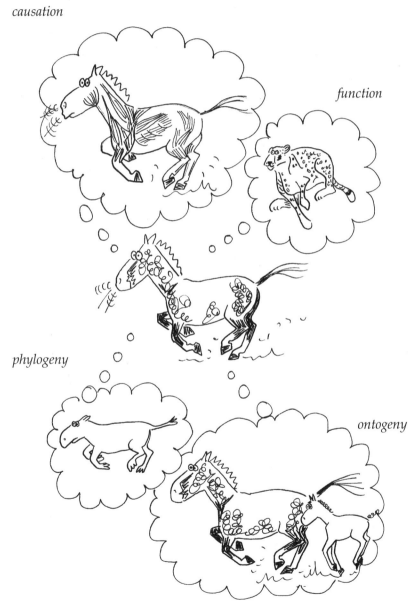

function

phylogeny

ontogeny

Fig. 1.1   Answers to Tinbergen's four questions.

but they are all correct. When asking ourselves 'why does ...?', we must appreciate that there are several different approaches and several answers. In order to understand behaviour fully we need to recognise and understand these four different approaches.

Ethology versus psychology

The study of behaviour therefore requires the application of several biological sciences. Traditionally these have been focussed into two broad overlapping disciplines, each with a different emphasis: ethology and psychology.

The early ethologists were mainly involved with the study of wild animals in their natural environment, believing that the forces of evolution had adapted the behaviour of animals. Ethologists, therefore, tended to concentrate on those aspects of behaviour which were inherited from one generation to the next, especially the genetic aspects of behaviour. Niko Tinbergen (1952) wrote: 'Learning and many other higher processes are secondary modifications of innate mechanisms.' To him and other early ethologists the nature of inherited behaviour was its most important feature.

Early psychologists, on the other hand, were more interested in the development of behaviour within the individual, and concentrated on trying to establish general and universal laws affecting behaviour and how it changes with learning. In this case one species of animal was often considered as good as another for modelling the general behaviour mechanisms of animals. They tended to emphasise the importance of the environment and nurturing. This is typified by the words of one of the most famous early psychologists, John Watson:

> 'Give me a dozen healthy infants, well formed, and my own specified world to bring them up in and I'll guarantee to take any one of them at random and train him to become any specialist I might select: doctor, lawyer, merchant, chief and yes, even beggar man and thief, regardless of his talents, peculiarities, tendencies, abilities, vocations and race of his ancestors.' (Watson 1913).

Because they were interested in different aspects of behaviour ethologists and psychologists had very different ways of studying it.

In the first half of the twentieth century furious arguments raged on the nature–nurture debate: psychologists demonstrated how flexible and changeable 'instinctive' behaviours were, and ethologists showed how animals would inherently respond to certain stimuli without learning. It is only as recently as the 1970s that the

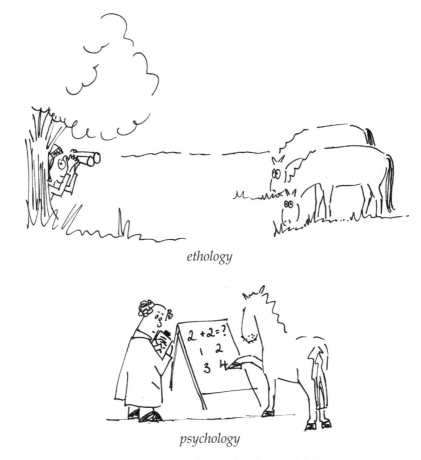

ethology

psychology

Fig. 1.2   Different approaches to the study of animal behaviour.

two sides really accepted that they were both making valid con-
tributions, and that most progress would be made if they put their
heads together.

The modern synthesis

The disciplines of psychology and ethology not only complement
each other well but are inextricably linked. You cannot have behaviour without both nature and nurture. Behaviour is the consequence of the constant interaction of genetic factors with the
environment; a process called epigenesis. Indeed, we could describe
behaviour as a phenotypic characteristic, just like size or coat colour. Unlike other phenotypic characteristics, however, behaviour is
variable on a day-to-day, or even a minute-by-minute basis.

McFarland (1993) suggests that the environment and genetics are
to behaviour what length and breadth are to a field. You cannot
have a field without both of these dimensions. We should resist the

temptation to talk about behaviour patterns being either genetic or learned, as if only one of these factors were important in determining behaviour. The combination of genetics and the environment sets the limits for the behaviour, just as length and breadth determine the boundaries of the field. They set the limits of an individual's ability and suggest certain predispositions. You would not go out and buy a Shetland pony from a children's farm if you had set your sights on getting round Badminton.

The constant remoulding of an animal's inherent behavioural tendencies by its environment is important from a training aspect. Horses do not just 'behave' because 'that's the way they are', they respond to their environment according to their abilities. In attempting to train the horse, we become part of its environment. This is a big responsibility, which we must be prepared to accept if we hope to be able to tap the horse's ability. We must make an effort to understand why a horse behaves in a particular way, and not just try to manipulate the results of the behaviour we see.

Techniques developed for studying behaviour in one discipline have also been borrowed by the other and resulted in great advances in our scientific understanding of behaviour. For example, the techniques used by psychologists to assess how animals respond to different rewards have been used to understand how animals naturally regulate their behaviour (see Kacelnik (1984) for experimental details). This has also helped us develop techniques to assess what is important for their well-being in captivity, as discussed in Chapter 10.

So what is behaviour?

We have already suggested that behaviour is a phenotypic feature, i.e. it is the result of the interaction between the environment and genetics at any given moment in time. We have also suggested that both the recent (proximate) and historical (ultimate) factors affecting it can be investigated. Recent factors include its immediate value and causation; historical factors include developmental issues. In both these cases behaviour is a means whereby an animal can adapt to its environment. In the short-term sense we can view behaviour as an external manifestation of internal physiology. A change is detected in the internal or external environments and this is processed by the animal which results in a change of behaviour. In order to understand behaviour, we must appreciate all these issues. With this understanding we are able to assess better how we manage horses and how we can improve. But first we must make sure that we study behaviour in a scientifically rigorous way.

A brief guide to conducting a behaviour study

The objective nature of data

Jennings, a behaviour physiologist, wrote in 1906,

> for those interested in the conscious aspects of behaviour, a presentation of the objective facts is a necessary preliminary to an intelligent discussion of the matter.

These words are not only applicable to conscious behaviour but also to any scientific study of animal behaviour. We all have our ideas as to why an animal does something in a particular way and what horses really get up to. The value of good science is that it allows us not only to offer an explanation of why something has occurred but also to predict why, when or how something is likely to recur. This means that we can prepare better for the future. Many people report their observations and feelings on all sorts of matters, but only if they are scientific can we really appreciate their true significance and compare them to other data. The scientific study of behaviour involves being as objective as possible about our observations. When we study behaviour we are interested in gathering data and this is the first of many problems we must overcome. Data are unbiased measurements. We can listen to a horse's heart and count the number of beats. The number we have is then a piece of data. If we report that the horse's heart seems a bit fast, this is not real data, but an interpretation of data. The horse may have recently run a race, have a fever, be a little nervous about us listening to its chest or just naturally have a higher than average heart rate. Only if we have more information can we interpret our data properly. It is therefore essential that we gather all the appropriate information in our study, before we discuss or try to interpret our results.

Descriptive and experimental studies

There are two broad types of behaviour study.

(1) There are those that describe and report what is happening, and so we have a record to which we may later wish to refer. This tells us what is happening in the world of horses.

(2) The second type of study is a form of experiment. We start with a question to which we want an answer. From this we think of a range of possible explanations. The aim then is to work out an experiment that would let us distinguish between them. We then gather our data and see which ideas we can discard. This does not mean that we have proved any that are left, since there may be other explanations which we had not thought of and which could not be disproved by the experiment. This is

an essential point in science which is commonly misunderstood. We do not go out to prove our ideas, we try to disprove all the alternatives.

A simple example will illustrate the point. Suppose we are interested in why horses crib-bite. We might suppose that horses do this in order to pass the time of day as there is little else for them to do in a stable (some might call this boredom). Alternatively, we might argue that they do it because they are very frustrated by being kept in the stable, particularly around meal times. At this time they can see their food but cannot get to it. We could possibly distinguish between these two explanations by giving a group of horses a toy containing food. This means that they have to work quite hard to get their ration. If the first explanation of cribbing is true then we might expect the amount of cribbing to go down when the toy is introduced. If cribbing is associated with frustration, then giving a horse a source of food which it cannot easily get to may be more frustrating. Horses are grazers and so may not be adapted to having to work for their food in the same way that a dog or cat has to. In this case we might expect the cribbing to get worse or stay the same but certainly not to get any better. An experiment somewhat similar to this has been done (Henderson *et al.* 1997). What they found was that some horses got better and others got worse. What does this tell us about why horses crib? Probably that there are several very different reasons why horses have this disturbing behaviour. Even if they had all responded the same way we could not say we now knew why horses crib. At best we could say why they probably do not.

Science can be very frustrating at times, but it can also be very exciting as you realise that there is so much that we still do not know. In this example the experimenters were measuring behaviour in order to test an idea, but whatever its purpose information needs to be gathered in a scientific manner.

Measurement

A horse's behaviour is a continuous process. As long as it is alive it is behaving. We can however divide behaviour into discrete units like galloping, chewing and kicking. When we use terms like these it may seem obvious to us what the horse is doing, but, as with any measure, like a metre, hand or second, we must ensure that we are using the term in a way which other people understand. If I say that my horse is 16 hands high then you know that it is 64 inches at the withers, even if the hand at the end of my wrist is five inches wide. That is because the term hand is defined as a four inch unit of measurement.

In behaviour there are few standard terms like the units of physics. We must therefore define the ones we use even if they seem obvious. Suppose I am interested in comparing the movement of horses around two different types of grassy paddock. I might use behaviour measures like walking, standing, trotting and grazing. Surely it is obvious what we mean by these terms? But when does grazing become standing or walking? If a horse takes three paces whilst moving to another clump of grass, is it walking or still grazing? If we say it is walking, is that the same behaviour as a horse that walks across the paddock to groom another horse? If not, then our measure is not recording anything meaningful. It is invalid.

'So what?' you might say, 'As long as I know what I've recorded, does it matter?' The answer to this in science is 'Yes: because if you can't tell me what you have measured I can't do my own study and compare results.' The value of your study is then at best limited to that experiment alone and at worst of no use at all. This could be because you were not as consistent as you thought. The definition lets everyone know exactly what you are recording and makes your observations into real data. We could test how consistent your observations are by videoing a bit of behaviour and asking you to record from it several times. If you have a good measure then you are likely to produce similar results each time. Your measure can then be said to be reliable.

So for good science our measures must be both valid and reliable. A valid measure describes only what it says it will and a reliable one is repeatable. These measures then form the basis of an ethogram. An ethogram is a catalogue of the behaviours performed by an animal. In an ideal world we would have a standard ethogram for all the behaviours which a horse can show, so that we have standard units of measurement as they do in physics. The gaits of the horse have been defined in this way (see Leach *et al.* 1984), and some good catalogues relating to specific types of behaviour have been produced like McDonnell and Haviland's ethogram of agonistic behaviour in a bachelor band (1995). Elsewhere we may have less published material which we can use or with which we can agree. We must therefore construct our own ethogram for most studies.

Behaviour can be measured at many different levels and the level we choose should be relevant to the study that we are undertaking. There is no point describing the position of every limb in the horse's body if we are only really interested in which gait it is using. When we have decided on our behavioural unit we need to consider the best way to define it. We could use a straightforward description such as:

Bite – opening and rapid closing of the jaws with the teeth grasping the flesh of another horse. The ears are laid back and lips retracted at this time.

Alternatively we could define the behaviours by means of an algorithm (flow diagram) such as that shown in Figure 1.3.

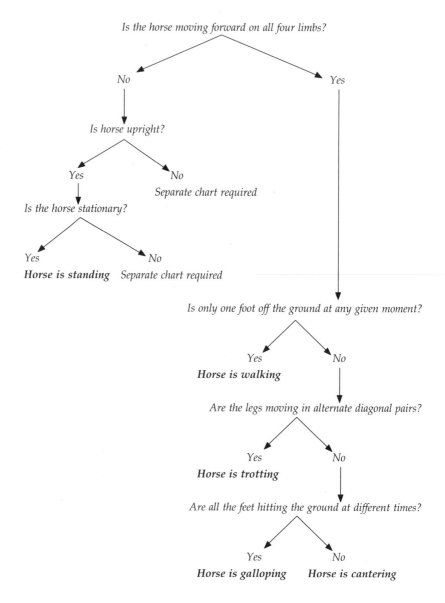

Fig. 1.3 Algorithm for identifying the normal gaits in the horse. Starting at the top of the page answer each question until you come to an explanation given in bold type.

When describing a behaviour in an ethogram, it is best if we keep to a description of what we can see and do not include any reference to function or motivation. The definition of bite given above is much better than 'attacking another horse with its mouth'. The problem with this last example is that we cannot know what is going on in another animal's head and so to depend on these factors means that we are more likely to have an unreliable measure.

Now we have decided on our units, what should we record? Once again we want to make sure that what we record is relevant. Some behaviours are 'events' like a bite, others are 'states' like walking. When we record events we are usually interested in whether or not they are occurring; in which case we will record how often they occur – their frequency. When we consider states, we may be interested in knowing not only whether it has occurred but also how long it went on for (duration). For behaviours which occur several times in short succession, such as mounting attempts by a stallion, we may be interested in the number of bouts of behaviour and number of instances within that bout (local rate) as well as its duration.

As well as scoring the horse's behaviour it may be useful to include some information about where or with whom it occurs, e.g. Barnaby bites Harry. Since there is a lot to record a shorthand is often used. In which case the last example may be recorded as 'B.b.H' for short. It is important to make sure that you can easily understand your shorthand and that it is unambiguous. If Barnaby butts Harry as well, we cannot use the same shorthand.

We now have the measures for the study. All we need to do now is decide how to use them in the study and to do this we must make two more decisions. We must choose our sampling technique and our recording technique.

◇ Sampling involves deciding what to watch.
◇ Recording involves when to write it all down.

Sampling techniques
There are four main types of sampling: ad libitum, focal, scan and behaviour.

(1) **Ad libitum sampling** This means you record as much as you can see at the given time. This is great in the early stages of a project when you want to get a feel of what is going on, or if some of the events that you are interested in are quite rare. The problem with this is that you will inevitably focus on certain types of behaviour (usually the most obvious ones) but can still easily gather a lot of useless information.

(2) **Focal sampling** With this technique you focus on a particular

unit in the field. This might be a specific horse, pair of horses or group of horses. With the additional help of video you may be able to focus on several groups, choosing one for each time you run through the video. This technique is useful if you are interested in what individuals are doing over a given time. An alternative way of doing this is to use the next technique.

(3) **Scan sampling** When you scan sample you observe the behaviour of different individuals in a set order, e.g. A then B then C then A then B etc. It means that you can cover more animals in less time but at the cost of some detail.

(4) **Behaviour sampling** This is used if you are interested in a specific behaviour, rather than the overall activity of an individual or group. You look out for the behaviour of interest and describe its context whenever it occurs in as much detail as required.

Recording techniques

When it comes to doing your observations you can either record behaviour the whole time or give yourself a break. There are therefore two broad categories of recording: continuous and intermittent.

(1) **Continuous recording** means that you can record the time, frequency, duration and latency for a behaviour accurately if necessary. The problem is that it is a lot of work and whilst you are recording you are bound to be missing some other information.

(2) **Intermittent recording** means that the data are recorded at fixed times. At this time we may decide that we are going to only record the behaviour that is happening at that instant (instantaneous recording), or we are going to record what has happened since the last instant (one zero recording). In either case, what we get is a collection of data relating to sample instants. We do not get real measure of duration, frequency, time or latency.

Consider the example in Figure 1.4. With continuous sampling we see six bouts of behaviour and may add the start and stop times of each. With 10 second instantaneous sampling we record three bouts, but can say nothing more. With 15 second instantaneous sampling we record no bouts of behaviour. With one zero sampling at 10 second intervals we appear to have nine bouts of behaviour.

The choice of technique can greatly effect the results obtained. Continuous recording is undoubtedly the most accurate if we need a lot of detail, but entails a lot of work. For comparative studies this

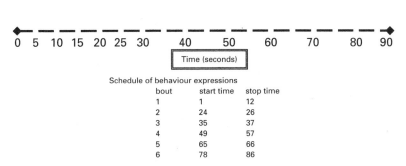

Fig. 1.4   The effect of sampling on the record obtained. See text for details.

extra work may not be necessary because we are interested in differences between groups. As long as we use the same rules for both populations and record enough data, the effect of any error should be the same in all the studies. In this case we do not have exact data but we still have useful data. If we are to use an intermittent recording technique, then we must think carefully about the time intervals that we use. This will depend on how long the behaviours in which we are interested last. If they are very short then short intervals or continuous sampling is necessary, but if the behaviour lasts for longer, then a greater interval is acceptable. If we hope to get an overall view of the activity of the animals in our study with intermittent sampling then we must recognise that this technique will bias the record towards those behaviours which last longer.

Conclusion

In summary, to conduct a good study:

(1)   Identify an area of interest
(2)   Ask a specific question about this which can be answered by gathering behavioural data
(3)   Design your study accordingly
(4)   Decide on your measures which should be valid, reliable and relevant
(5)   Pilot your study and revise the protocol accordingly
(6)   Gather your data
(7)   Analyse your data
(8)   Assess the implications of your data in the light of its limitations
(9)   Draw your conclusions.

TOPICS FOR DISCUSSION

◇ What are the advantages and disadvantages of physical descriptions of behaviour compared to functional descriptions of equine behaviour?

◇ Discuss the causative, ontogenic, phylogenic and functional factors that might be involved in explaining why a horse neighs, shies or refuses to jump a wall.

◇ What are the advantages of the scientific method over casual observation in equine behaviour studies?

◇ Is behaviour just physiology?

◇ Discuss the concepts of reliability and validity in behaviour studies.

◇ Consider the decisions which have to be made at each stage of a specific study of the behaviour of horses and how you would justify each choice.

◇ When might a descriptive study of horse behaviour be more useful than an experimentally based one?

References and further reading

Alcock, J. (1993) *Animal Behaviour: an evolutionary approach.* Sinauer Associates Inc., Sunderland, USA.

Goodenough, J., McGuire, B. & Wallace, R. (1993) *Perspectives on Animal Behaviour.* J. Wiley & Sons, New York.

Halliday, T.R. & Slater, P.J.B. (1983) *Animal Behaviour.* Blackwell Scientific Publications, Oxford.

Henderson, J. V., Waran, N.K. & Young, R.J. (1997) Behavioural enrichment for horses: the effect of a foraging device (the 'Equiball') on the performance of stereotypic behaviour in stabled horses. In: *Proceedings of the First International Conference on Veterinary Behavioural Medicine*, eds Mills, D.S., Heath, S.E. & Harrington, L.J., UFAW, Potters Bar.

Hinde, R.A. (1970) *Animal Behaviour.* McGraw-Hill, New York.

Houpt, K.A. (1991) *Domestic Animal Behavior for Veterinarians and Animal Scientists.* Iowa State University Press, USA.

Jennings, H.S. (1906) *The Behaviour of Lower Organisms.* Colombia University Press, New York.

Kacelnik, A. (1984) Central place foraging in Starlings (*Sturnus vulgaris*). Part I. Patch residence time. *Journal of Animal Ecology*, **53**, 283–299.

Krebs, J.R. & Davies, N.B. (1996) *An Introduction to Behavioural Ecology.* Blackwell Science, Oxford.

Manning, A. & Dawkins, M.S. (1992) *An Introduction to Animal Behaviour.* Cambridge University Press, Cambridge.

Martin, P. & Bateson, P. (1993) *Measuring Behaviour, An Introductory Guide.* 2nd edn. Cambridge University Press, Cambridge.

McDonnell, S.M. & Haviland, J.C.S. (1995) *Agonistic ethogram of the equid bachelor band.* Applied Animal Behaviour Science **43**, 147–188.

McFarland, D.(1993) *Animal Behaviour*. Longman Scientific and Technical, Harlow.

Sparks, J. (1983) *The Discovery of Animal Behaviour*. W. Collins Sons & Co Ltd., Glasgow.

Tinbergen, N. (1952) 'Derived' activities, their causation, biological significance, origin and emancipation during evolution. *Quarterly Review of Biology* **27**, 1–32.

Toates, F.M. (1980) *Animal Behaviour. A Systems Approach*. John Wiley & Sons, Chichester.

Watson, J.B. (1914) Psychology as the behaviorist views it. *Psychological Review* **20**, 158–177.

2. *Origins of Behaviour*

An evolutionary approach to understanding behaviour

The theory of evolution proposes how modern day life has come to be and how it might change in the future. Often, when we first think of evolution, we see it as a way of explaining how we are all related and how our bodies have adapted from common ancestors or structures. The evidence is in the fossil record. But evolutionary theory has far more to offer than this; it explains how both structure and behaviour are related to the environment. It is the same process which brings about changes in both of these and so understanding it is an essential foundation to the explanation of behaviour.

Remember Tinbergen's four questions in the last chapter? Any interpretation of why a horse performs a certain behaviour should have a sound 'evolutionary' explanation. If it does not, then either evolutionary theory is wrong, or our interpretation is wrong. Since there is now quite a substantial amount of evidence to support the theory of evolution, there is a good chance that, if we cannot explain how a behaviour could have possibly evolved within this framework, then it is our interpretation of the behaviour that is wrong.

Behaviour leaves no fossil remains but is related to the living structures and environmental conditions that do leave physical evidence behind. On this basis we may be able to infer some of the behavioural foundations of the horse which are as much a part of its make up as the fundamental structure on which its anatomy is built.

In summary then, understanding evolution in the horse is essential because:

(1) The theory of evolution provides a framework within which we can check and test our interpretations of behaviour to see if they can possibly be right.
(2) It helps us to appreciate the behavioural foundations on which the behaviour characteristics of a group of horses or individual are built.

(3) It highlights the relationship between form and function, which can cause so many welfare, management and performance problems if it is ignored.

(4) It emphasises the distinction between those traits which might respond to selective breeding and those which are unlikely to do so.

In this chapter we will concentrate on the first of these, the process of evolution. In the next chapter we will build on this theme and illustrate these processes in action during the prehistory of the horse. This will provide the basis for understanding the further points which are discussed throughout the rest of the book.

Lamarck versus Darwin

Evolution is the change which occurs to an organism during its long-term developmental (phylogenetic) history. Evolution does not drive change, it merely describes the changes which occur. In the nineteenth century, there were two main theories as to how evolution might occur.

Lamarckian theory

The first was described by Lamarck in 1809 in his *Philosophie Zoologique*. He suggested that features which developed within the lifetime of an individual as a result of need or effort could be passed on from one generation to another. For example, if horses were required to eat food from a great height, then the constant effort to reach up might result in horses developing longer necks and front legs. This feature would then develop over a number of generations. Horses would then start to look like giraffes. This reason for such a change occurring is no longer recognised as credible within the scientific community. If we accepted Lamarckian theory, it should follow that breeding from race winners would produce faster and faster horses all the time, as faster parents will produce faster offspring. This is not the case.

Darwinian theory

Charles Darwin and Alfred Russel Wallace proposed the main alternative explanation as to why horses might evolve into giraffe-like creatures in this situation. It is often forgotten that it was only when Wallace came to the same conclusions as Darwin that Darwin was encouraged to write down his ideas. Darwin noticed the following factors.

(1) **Variability** We are all different, i.e. there is variation within any population of individuals.

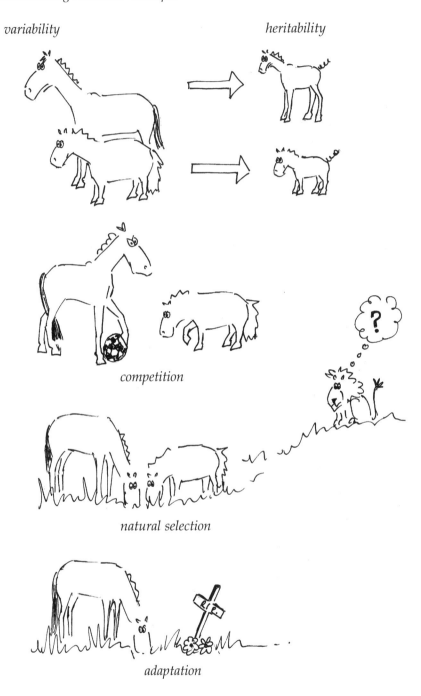

variability   *heritability*

competition

natural selection

adaptation

Fig. 2.1   Darwin noticed variability, heritability, competition, natural selection and adaptation.

(2) **Heritability** We can pass on certain traits to our offspring, i.e. some features are heritable.

(3) **Competition** More individuals are born than the world can support, i.e. there is competition to survive.

(4) **Natural selection** Environmental pressures affect some individuals more than others and so it is not completely random as to who lives and who dies.

(5) **Adaptation** Those individuals that live longest will leave most offspring carrying their heritable traits. So over generations the population will change to reflect the features of those best adapted to the environment, i.e. adaptive evolution will occur as a result of natural selection.

Adaptation

In the example above, some horses living where grass is in short supply, which happen to have the longest necks, are able to eat more and so produce more offspring which tend to be more similar to their parents than their short-necked relatives.

To use a more serious example which highlights a common confusion, the horse did not develop longer legs so that it could escape predators, but rather those with long legs escaped predators and passed this trait on, whilst their shorter legged friends got eaten. Eventually there comes a point when the benefits of longer legs (such as a longer stride) are outweighed by the costs (e.g. the effectiveness of the muscle required to move them, the tendency for the limbs to break down, etc.). In this way, an optimal position is reached until another trait happens to arise which allows the development of an alternative strategy.

The development of longer legs was a consequence of the environment, not a deliberate adaptation to it.

Altruism: a threat to Darwinian logic

Altruism describes an entirely selfless action which shows concern for the welfare of others, and may even result in the death of the selfless individual, for instance a mother protecting her young, or a healthy animal refusing to leave an injured companion in danger.

If Darwin's theory is correct, individuals should always be selfish, since this maximises their reproductive potential and their chances of survival (individual fitness). Obviously this is not the case, as we see many examples of altruism within the animal kingdom. This anomaly obviously posed a threat to our neat Darwinian theory. Natural selection was all very well, but what was really being selected?

Genes, not individuals

A hundred years after the original theory of natural selection, a modified version was proposed which incorporated what is now known about genetics and heredity. It was recognised that natural selection did not occur at the level of the individual but at the level of the gene. The individual is merely a vehicle for the gene, providing a means by which the gene can produce more copies of itself. This is what Dawkins meant when he referred to 'the selfish gene', in his book of the same name.

Darwin's idea was not wrong, but his theory needed to be applied at the genetic level rather than at the level of the individual. It is now as follows:

(1)   **Variation** The gene that codes for a particular trait comes in many forms, and these forms are known as alleles. This underlies the variation that is seen in the population. The fewer the alleles, the less variation there is.

(2)   **Heredity** During the process of sexual reproduction, alleles are passed from both parents to their offspring, i.e. we inherit traits from our parents.

(3)   **Competition** The genes to which alleles relate are found at a precise position (locus) on the chromosome. There are therefore a limited number of places available within any individual. If an animal is diploid, it has one chromosome from each parent and so two loci are available for the four alleles possessed by the parents. There is therefore competition for places and not every form of the allele will necessarily be passed on.

(4)   **Natural selection** Any allele which gives an advantage to its own replication and survival, e.g. by increasing the reproductive capacity of the individual which carries it, will persist in the population at the expense of other alleles.

(5)   **Adaptation** The composition of the gene pool then changes with time as a reflection of the advantage (fitness) that particular genes convey in a given environment.

Maximising genetic potential by acts of altruism

There are three reasons why a horse may not be completely selfish.

Kin selection

In 1964, Hamilton proposed that animals should be viewed as a collection of genes, and therefore they can be expected to behave in a way which maximises their genetic potential, rather than their individual potential. He suggested that in order to maximise their genetic potential (or inclusive fitness), animals may sometimes behave unselfishly at the individual level. This way, the gene increases its potential in certain circumstances by acts of altruism. Take the following example; a mother with four offspring is attacked by a predator. The situation is such that either she or all her offspring will be killed. The mother constitutes 100% maternal genetic material, each offspring has half of its genetic material from its mother, and half from the father. Since there are four offspring, together they carry 4 × 50% of the mother's genetic material, amounting to 200%.

If the offspring are likely to survive to breed successfully, altruism on the mother's part makes perfect selfish sense at the genetic level (particularly if she is so old that she is unlikely to breed again) since the loss of the mother and her genes is only half the genetic loss which would occur if her offspring were to die instead. Genes which encourage altruism towards genetically related individuals in these sorts of circumstance may therefore persist. This gives us another example of natural selection. John Maynard Smith (1969) called this process kin selection.

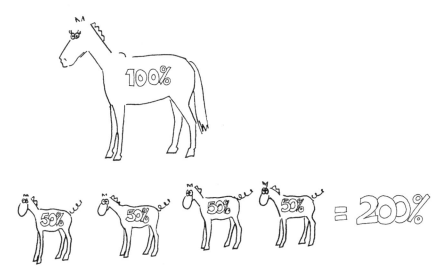

Fig. 2.2 A mother may represent less of her own genetic material than her offspring.

Reciprocal altruism

Not all altruistic behaviour involves suicide or sacrifice for the sake of a relative. Trivers (1971) suggested that altruistic behaviour could evolve in individuals if it involved little cost and the favour was directed to individuals likely to return it later. This would work as long as opportunities to repay the debt occurred quite frequently, and as long as individuals could recognise each other. Such animals would also need to have the mental ability to memorise events and individuals. This behaviour is known as reciprocal altruism and is only likely to be seen in social species with a strong tendency to co-operate. The horse has such tendencies, and, as we see in later chapters, we depend heavily on its co-operation for successful management. It sometimes seems to show such behaviour, but we do not know for sure whether it really has the right sort of brain and perception abilities.

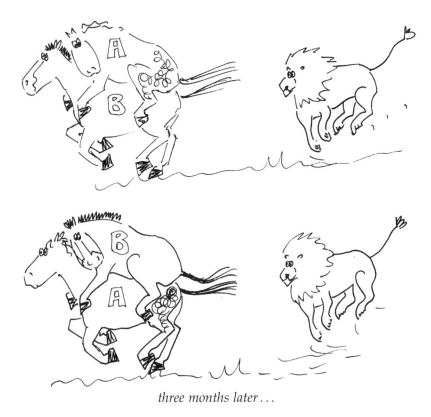

three months later . . .

Fig. 2.3 Reciprocal altruism.

Helpers at the nest
Sometimes altruistic behaviour occurs in animals when they are neither a relative of the individual helped nor likely to have the help repaid. For example, some animals help others to rear their off-spring. Helpers at the nest (as they are known) may not benefit directly from any of the individuals that they help. This is certainly a sacrifice on their part, so why do they bother? It seems that they still gain in the long (genetic) run, since such helpers tend to be

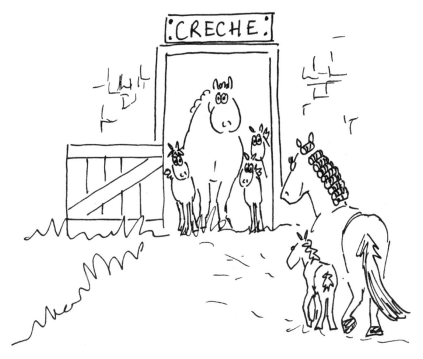

Fig. 2.4 Helping others rear their offspring may make you a better mother when it is your turn.

more successful when it comes to rearing their own offspring. It's better to experiment with motherhood on someone else's baby first!

Group selection: a flawed theory

In 1964 Wynne Edwards proposed a different solution to the problem of altruism. His idea was known as group selection.

He suggested that the genes within an individual may guide it to behave altruistically for the good of the species. He thought that if individuals of a given species were entirely selfish they would breed so much that there would be a population explosion. This would then lead to widespread starvation and the annihilation of the species. There is a certain attraction to this idea and the theory is often heard repeated when people try to explain phenomena like the 'helpers at the nest'. The helpers are helping the success of the species.

There is however, a critical flaw to this theory as Williams (1966) pointed out. Suppose such a trait did exist. What would happen if a mutation arose which caused selfishness? Who would be more successful? What then happens to the population over time? The answer is that the selfish ones take over. Group selection might

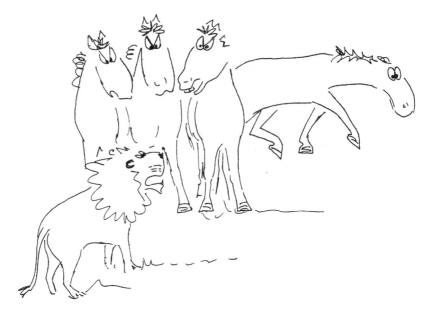

Fig. 2.5 Explanations for behaviour based on individuals acting for the good of the group do not work when cheats are better off.

possibly occur in very special circumstances, for example amongst isolated populations in which there is also a low rate of genetic mutation, but, it does not apply to any known horse populations.

Evolutionary throwbacks and genetic jumps

Occasionally genetic throwbacks occur, for instance a horse being born with multiple toes. This phenomenon is called 'atavism'. If we know that genes code for specific protein molecules, it may seem surprising that such large mutations can occur. The answer lies in the fact that some genes are able to regulate the activity of a whole group of others. These are known as 'regulatory' genes. If a mutation occurs in one of these, activities which were previously repressed, may be switched on. Imagine that there is a gene which prevents more than one toe being present per foot. This could lead to a population of animals with single toes. If a mutation occurred in this regulatory gene, individuals could exist with more than one toe, i.e. throwbacks could occur. This is what seems to happen in reality. Species tend to share a lot of genetic material with other species, and their differences come not only from having unique genes, but also from repressing some of those that are shared.

This example of throwbacks demonstrates the way that evolution can occur not only on a very gradual basis, but also in quite large, rapid jumps. The fossil record of the horse certainly seems to show a process that involved bursts of large and rapid changes as well as periods of more gradual change. We can therefore think of evolution as a punctuated process of adaptation.

Adaptation and apparent stupidity in domestic horses

So evolution is the consequence of a continuous process of adaptation to the environment. It can only occur if genetic mutants arise in the population, giving variety from which natural selection can occur.

What sort of traits are advantageous to an individual? They can be broadly divided into three groups:

(1) **Exploitation traits** Those that allow an animal to compete more effectively for essential resources such as food and mates. These are traits which improve exploitation of the environment.

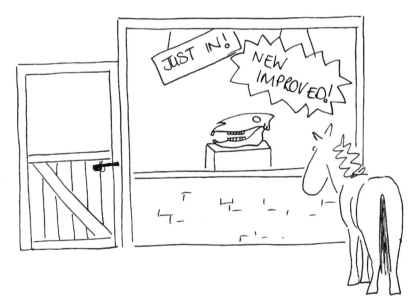

Fig. 2.6 Traits which allow exploitation of a new environment will be favoured by natural selection.

(2) **Survival traits** Those that allow an animal to survive in the continual contest between predator and prey. Some authors , e.g. Krebs and Davies (1993), call this an evolutionary arms race, because if an animal develops a trait which gives it a better chance of escaping its predators, then soon, only those

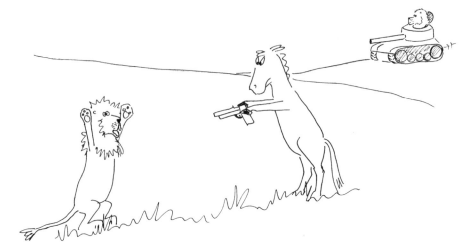

Fig. 2.7   There is a constant arms race between predator and prey.

> with this trait will be left in the population. There is then intense selective pressure on the predators, and only the best hunters will survive.

One of the trends that tends to be seen, unless there are particular environmental pressures against it, is a steady increase in body size over the evolutionary history of a species. This is known as Cope's Law.

(3)   **Sexual selection traits** Some traits increase the attractiveness of an individual to members of the opposite sex. These are usually associated with emphasising the animal's fitness or performance. Since they are preferred mates they will leave more offspring and so the population will change to emphasise these traits in a process known as sexual selection. Sexual selection helps to explain why the males and females of a

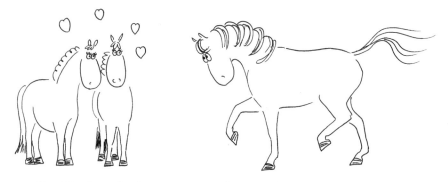

Fig. 2.8   Sexual selection occurs when certain traits in one sex encourage the opposite sex to reproduce with them.

species look and behave differently. Some of the behaviours which develop as a result of this process, such as that of the courting stallion, can seem quite spectacular or bizarre. We will discuss the importance of these signals of fitness and their relevance to horse behaviour in Chapter 8 on reproductive behaviour.

From evolutionary theory we can predict that lifetime behaviour strategies will develop which will tend to maximise the genetic transmission to future generations, but this is a long-term consequence of many shorter term strategies. An animal cannot know the ultimate consequences that every potential behaviour will have on its long-term reproductive fitness, and so its immediate behaviour will be governed by the rules of thumb that, over evolutionary time scales, tend to produce maximum return in the long term.

The captive horse is still largely a vehicle for its pre-domestication genes and so can be expected to follow the same rules even though the current environment and consequences differ radically from those in which they originally developed. In the light of this, it is hardly any wonder that the behaviour of the domestic horse may at times seem inappropriate or 'stupid', but in an evolutionary sense he is like a fish out of water. This is an important point to remember when we are trying to assess the behaviour of the domestic horse.

Evolution and the variety of behaviour

Earlier we said that any allele that gives an advantage to its own replication and survival would persist in the population, but what if no single trait is consistently more effective? Various forms of alleles will exist, and we will see a variety of physical forms of an individual. This is known as polymorphism.

Similarly, there may be several different behavioural strategies for dealing with the same problem, each of them genetically determined but some of which are more likely to be effective for an individual.

The range of tactics which yields the maximum return when occurring at a certain frequency represents the point of equilibrium for the situation and is called the evolutionary stable strategy. For example; there are various ways that a stallion could maximise his reproductive potential in a given environment, with the effectiveness of each depending on his physical characteristics.

Strategy 1: Protect a harem of several mares from all other stallions This is fine if you are a mature, strong stallion but not if you are younger, smaller or weaker. Deliberately picking a fight with a large strong stallion to try and win his mares would probably not be very good for your genes.

Strategy 2: Try and find a harem without a resident stallion This might occur occasionally but a harem is rarely left unattended. A stallion may leave the group after he has been defeated, but then usually the winner of the fight has already taken up residence. An older stallions may also take on an understudy which inherits the group when he dies. The chances, therefore, of finding an available group of females on their own are pretty small.

Strategy 3: Join up with males in similar circumstances If it comes across a harem, the bachelor group as a whole may provide sufficient distraction for the resident stallion to allow one of them to sneak in and mate with a mare.

Strategy 4: Live alone, but quite close to a harem You are then in a position to just sneak in when the stallion is not paying full attention.

Strategy 1 would be the obvious choice, but is only an option for the strongest stallions. Strategies 2 to 4 are not as efficient as defending your own harem, but as long as they work some of the time the trait could be passed on, albeit at a lower rate. All three of these

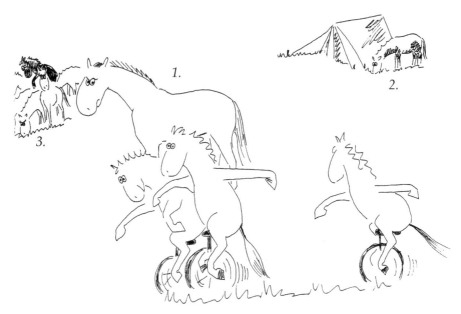

Fig. 2.9   Games theory predicts that when no one single strategy is always a winner, then a number of different strategies may exist in the population.
Strategy 1 – protect a harem of mares
Strategy 2 – wait until a harem is free
Strategy 3 – sneak in while the boss is distracted.

strategies can exist within a population, as each may give an advantage in a certain situation.

The idea that when there is no one sure-fire way to win in the game of life we will see different rules for different individuals was first proposed by Maynard Smith (1974) and called 'Games Theory'. Everyone plays according to their strengths and, as long as you are likely to be successful sooner or later, your genes will survive.

Conclusion

Together these are the processes which underpin the evolution of the horse. As a result we see the animal of today, an individual which is well adapted to its original lifestyle in both form and behaviour. This is the animal which we must work with in order to start to understand its behaviour. These processes help us to appreciate the limits and nature of the changes that have occurred. In the next chapter we will look at the evolutionary history of the horse in more detail. We will see how the nature of the horse as a species is built upon a succession of irreversible changes which occurred for many important reasons. This then sets limits to the adaptability of the individual within its lifetime.

TOPICS FOR DISCUSSION

◇ Are horses as a species ever likely to adapt to the stress of confinement and isolation if we keep them housed in stables for enough generations?

◇ With all the efforts being made to improve bloodstock, why are races being won with much the same time as a hundred years ago?

◇ Does altruism really exist?

◇ Compare and contrast behavioural traits which have helped the horse to survive against pressure from predators, with those that have increased attractiveness between individuals.

◇ If we kept breeding for larger, faster horses what factors are likely to limit progress?

◇ What potential problems is the domestic horse likely to encounter which are never faced by its free-living relatives? How can it adapt to these?

◇ Consider the factors which help explain the variation seen in equine behaviour strategies directed towards a specific goal, e.g. rearing young.

References and further reading

Darwin, C. (1859) *On the Origin of Species.* Murray, London.

Dawkins, R. (1976) *The Selfish Gene.* Oxford University Press, Oxford.

Dennett, D.C. (1995) *Darwin's Dangerous Idea.* Penguin, London.

Hamilton W.D. (1964) The genetical evolution of social behaviour. *Journal of Theoretical Biology* **7**, 1–52.

Krebs, J.R. & Davies, N.B. (1993) *An Introduction to Behavioural Ecology.* Blackwell Science, Oxford.

Maynard Smith, J. (1964) *Evolution and the Theory of Games.* Cambridge University Press. Cambridge.

Trivers, R.I. (1971) The evolution of reciprocal altruism, *Quarterly Review of Biology* **46**, 31–7.

Williams, G.C. (1966) *Adaptation and Natural Selection.* Princeton University Press, Princeton.

Wilson, E.O. (1975) *Sociobiology: The New Synthesis.* Belknap Press, Harvard.

Wynne Edwards, D.C. (1986) *Evolution through Group Selection.* Blackwell Scientific Publications, Oxford.

3. *The Evolutionary History of the Horse*

Introduction

The horse offers one of the most complete fossil histories, and is consequently frequently cited as a 'typical example' of evolution. The story is often told as if the horse was constantly improving itself; from the first, very primitive horse, *Hyracotherium* (formerly known as *Eohippus*), to today's supreme athlete, *Equus*. In fact, each evolutionary distinct individual existed because it was well adapted to its environment at the time. If it was not for the fact that the world kept changing, *Hyracotherium* would still be around, and we would have nothing to ride!

During the evolution of the horse, the position of the great land masses on the globe has changed enormously, with continents breaking apart and colliding on an occasional basis. There have also been enormous climatic changes which have heralded the mass extinction of species and groups which did not adapt both physi-cally and behaviourally. The ancestry of the horse has been subjected to similar stresses and, if it had not been for a few coincidences, the horse would have been wiped out along with many other prehistoric lines. The evolutionary history of the horse is a fascinating saga of fortunate survival, as we shall see, but first we shall consider some of the general changes that have occurred in its history.

Evolutionary trends in the horse

Evolution is progressive, constantly building on what has gone before but not reversing its steps except for occasional 'throwback' mutations in individuals. As a result we tend to see certain general trends throughout the evolutionary history of a species. In the horse we see development of the following themes:

(1) Increase in body size.
(2) Development and specialisation of the brain, in particular, an

expanded neocortex – an area concerned with learning and the
processing of sensory information.

(3) Decrease in the number of functional toes.
(4) Loss of toe pads and development of hooves.
(5) Relative lengthening of the limbs compared to the body.
(6) Fusion of some of the lower limb bones.
(7) Development of specialised locomotor systems which increase
the efficiency of certain gaits.

All of these have given horses an advantage in the evolutionary
'arms race' described in the previous chapter. In particular they
have allowed a relatively large animal to be quite fast for its size and
weight. If you are big, only big predators can eat you, and if you are
fast they will have to be quick too. This narrows down the field of
potential threats.

Other traits enabled the horse to exploit more efficiently the large
grasslands which began to appear 50 million years ago. These
included:

(1) Development of long lasting, high crowned teeth (hypsodonty)
with a larger grinding surface area.
(2) Elongation of the muzzle, which allows the retention of the
maximum number of functioning block-like teeth.
(3) Development of hind-gut fermentation.
(4) Development of regions of the neocortex of the brain associated with the processing of increased sensory input from the
lips and mouth, which allows more selective browsing and
grazing habits.

We can therefore expect the horse's maintenance behaviours to be
refined towards maximising the efficiency of grazing over long
periods of time.

Figure 3.1 shows a classic evolutionary tree for the horse. The
many branches show how the families are related and this sort of
diagram is preferable to those which show evolution along a 'time-
line' such as that shown in Figure 3.2. Each branch represents a
clade, or a large family of related species.

More recently, greater emphasis has been put on the development of certain key characteristics for the classification of individuals. This can be represented as shown in Figure 3.3. Since every
species is named at the same level, it helps to emphasise the point
that it is not inevitable that a species will evolve into another
improved version which will supersede it, a process known as
orthogenesis. Each species was good in its day.

Although Figure 3.3 shows the development of physical
characteristics, it is likely that certain key behaviours occur in

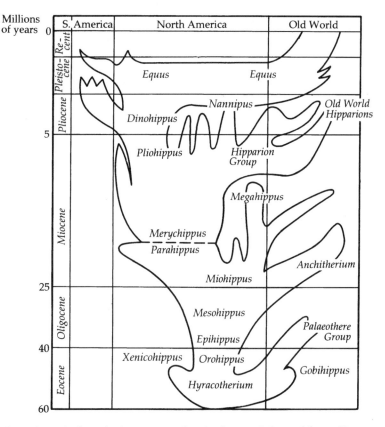

Fig. 3.1   A typical evolutionary tree for the horse. Adapted from Simpson (1951), *Horses: The Story of the Horse Family in the Modern World and through Sixty Million Years of History*, OUP, Oxford, and MacFadden (1992) *Fossil Horses: Systematics, Palaeobiology and Evolution of the Family Equidae*, CUP, Cambridge. Dashed line represents development of grazing rather than browsing lifestyle.

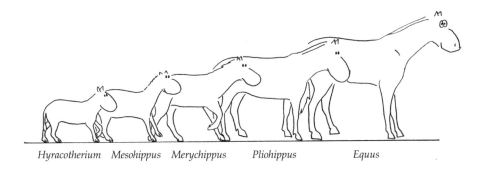

Fig. 3.2   Time-line diagram illustrating the evolutionary 'descent' of the horse.

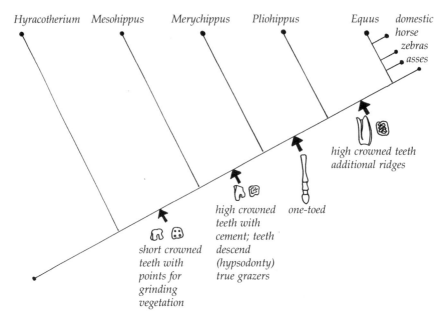

Fig. 3.3   Cladogram for the evolution of the horse. Adapted from
MacFadden (1992), *Fossil Horses, Systematics, Palaeobiology, and Evolution of
the Family Equidae*, CUP, Cambridge.

association with some of these, such as the move from browsing to
grazing or the development of specific gaits. Sometimes behaviour
and form are inextricably linked and we may have problems when
we seek to separate them in the domestic environment, as we shall
see later.

Classification of horses

The study of the classification of things is known as taxonomy.
There are many ways in which we could classify animals, we could
for example classify all animals with wings together in which case
the bat and the sparrow would be in the same group. The problem
with this technique is that it lumps animals together which only
share one or a few arbitrary characteristics in common.

Phylogeny

In the light of evolutionary theory, it would make more sense to
classify animals together on the basis of their evolutionary history
(phylogeny). Animals would then be grouped together on the basis
of how near their closest ancestor is. Common ancestors then become
the root of a division. This is a rule which can be applied consistently
to divide up several different levels of group. This allows the
development of a hierarchical classification, with members of the
lower levels sharing more physical and behavioural characteristics.

Unfortunately it is at this level that there is most confusion as different authors have used different features at different times to determine the division between different groups of animals. Nevertheless using this system we can represent the taxonomy of the domestic horse as shown below. The first word indicates the level of classification, whilst the part in italics shows to which group at this level the horse belongs:

Kingdom – *Animals* This is the highest level of division, all animals share certain cellular features which are not found amongst plants, fungi, or micro-organisms.

Phylum – *Chordates* All chordates are animals and have at least the primitive basis of a backbone at some stage of their development. It therefore excludes groups of animals like insects, worms and sponges.

Class – *Mammals* All mammals produce milk for their young to suckle. They also tend to have the potential to grow hair and most do not lay eggs but develop the young inside the body of the mother. A process known as vivipary. We can therefore exclude animals like birds and reptiles at this point, but recognise that the horse has more in common with them than it does with insects and the others excluded earlier.

Order – *Perissodactyl* These are all mammals with an odd number of toes which have hooves (ungulates). It suggests that the horse has more in common with the rhinoceros and tapir that it has with the hippopotamus, human, antelope or cow.

Family – *Equidae* This includes all the breeds of horse, the various species of zebra, the asses and the donkeys. The first distinct ancestor of the equidae was *Hyracotherium* formerly known as *Eohippus*, the dawn horse.

Genus – *Equus* Some authors have proposed a separate genus (*Asinus*) for the donkey and ass. This would emphasise the belief that the domestic horse is more closely related to the zebra and extinct species like the quagga than it is to these other species. However many authors maintain that all of these species belong to the same genus.

Species – *Caballus* This brings together all the various breeds of domestic horse. Species are sometimes divided further into sub-species or breeds. Przewalski's horse, the Mongolian wild horse, is described as a separate species of *Equus* in some texts, but is more commonly described as a sub-species of *Equus caballus* or *Equus ferus* (the term used by some authors to distinguish the wild horse from its domestic form). Members of the same species are capable of breeding together to produce fertile offspring. When referring to a species it is normal practice to use both the genus (or generic name) spelt with a capital letter, and the specific name, without a capital.

The sub-species may also be given after this. All of these words are written in italics or underlined and are usually derived from some Latin term. So the true name for the domestic horse is *Equus caballus caballus* and that for Przewalski's horse is *Equus ferus przewalskii* or *Equus caballus przewalskii*. This might seem a bit long winded but it is much more precise and less confusing than simply using the term 'horse' which might refer to anything within the family of equidae.

The precision of the system is its main attraction to science, even if there is dispute over the preferred terminology.

There may be good reason to distinguish between the wild and domestic forms of an animal since, as we shall see, the selective processes associated with domestication may result in significant physical and behavioural differences between the two forms. However it is important to realise that the behavioural patterns associated with the domestic species are built upon the behaviours provided by millions of years in the wild and many of these cannot be simply wiped out by a bit of selective breeding. If we ignore this, then the horse is likely to be the one that suffers. Some fundamental features are determined early in the evolutionary history of a species and are reflected in their widespread distribution among the various related taxa.

Such features cannot easily be changed even in captivity. For example, the herbivorous nature of the horse was determined early on and subsequent evolution has developed and refined the system physically and behaviourally towards its diet. Just as the horse is not likely to be able to survive on a carnivorous diet, it is unlikely to adapt well to other foods which differ radically in form from its natural diet. As we will see later (see Chapter 10) this might include a diet based on concentrates but this does not mean that the 'natural way' is the only way as flexibility is an integral part of the system.

Early evolution of the horse

We will now trace the pre-historical basis to some of the behaviour patterns associated with the modern horse.

The ancestor of all modern mammalian herbivores

Around the Cretaceous–Tertiary period, between 70 and 65 million years ago, an order of animals appeared known as condylarths. These included the ancestors of all modern day mammalian herbivores. They were relatively unspecialised, with five toes on each foot and the maximum number of teeth found in mammals, i.e. six incisors, two canines, eight premolars and six molars in both the upper and lower jaws. The cheek teeth (molars and premolars) were fairly square in cross section and each had four primary cusps which helped to grind the vegetation which made up its diet. From this point on, it would take more change than could occur by chance for there to be a radical switch in feeding preference. So the horse is first and foremost a herbivorous mammal with associated behaviours.

The ancestor of odd-toe ungulates

A family within the condylarths, known as the phenacodontids, was the ancestor of all modern day perissodactyls. By the Palaeocene, one generic form, *Phenacodus*, had appeared in North America while it was still connected to the Eurasian continent. Some species were very similar to the early forms of *Hyracotherium* and looked a bit like a small elongated hairy pig, with a long tail and padded toes (Figure 3.4). The upper and lower parts of the limb were of similar length. None of the limb bones were fused which allowed the limbs to rotate. The eyes were close to the mid-line of the head and pointed forward. In total the animal was about 1.7 metres long. It was no great athlete but then there was less pressure from carnivores and an abundance of vegetation. So it could survive in various forms amongst the extensive woodlands of the time with enough success to spread widely through the land mass.

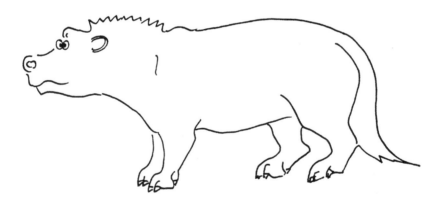

Fig. 3.4   *Phenacodus* was a pig-like ancestor of the horse.

Hyracotherium

During the Eocene period between 55 and 39 million years ago, there was quite a dramatic change in the climate. There was less rainfall and large grasslands began to appear, resulting in a patchwork of woodland and savannah over large areas of land in the northern hemisphere. This provided new opportunities for those species which could take advantage of it. One such individual was *Hyracotherium*. This was a small creature, only 0.5 metres high at most to the shoulder. It had padded feet with four hoofed toes on the fore foot and three behind. It had a stiff arched back and could probably trot, canter and gallop like a horse. *Hyracotherium* was a browser, living on the soft shoots and leaves of trees and other plants, which are a higher quality forage than grass. These food-stuffs were also far more abundant in the environment of the time. *Hyracotherium* was hugely successful, and fossil specimens have been found in both Europe and North America.

Adaptive radiation

When a species succeeds in taking advantage of a new environ-ment, there is a population explosion as there is little competition initially. The larger the number of individuals the greater the number of mutations in any given period of time. Since the new environment is not yet saturated with competitors or predators, there is a greater chance that some of these mutated individuals may be able survive in new, under-exploited niches. This new population will then become the focus of attention of predators, who may drive the selection for even better adaptation to this niche and predator avoidance, both physically and behaviourally. As a result, an initial coloniser is responsible for the rise of a whole variety of species with different traits and behaviour tendencies. This process is referred to as 'divergent evolution'. In this case each species is adapted to a different niche and the consequence is the 'adaptive radiation' of the group.

New species: new opportunity or new threat?

The emergence of a new species does not necessarily herald the extinction of its ancestor. This will depend upon how well adapted an individual is to the current environment. A new species does not have to be a replacement, it may just be an alternative form. If the environment changes, one sort may prove to be better adapted. For example, in North America *Hyracotherium* gave rise to a number of genera including *Gobihippus* and *Xenicohippus* which became extinct while *Hyracotherium* was still about (see Fig. 3.1). However in Eurasia *Hyracotherium* gave rise to a whole group of genera, collectively known as the palaeotheres. These species seemed to be more successful and over the course of a few million years replaced *Hyracotherium* in this part of the world. But with a continuing fall in global temperature through the next epoch of time (the Oligocene), less rainfall and an associated change in the vegetation, this group was no longer so well adapted and further adaptations did not arise. As a result, disaster struck – all the palaeotheres died out.

Since Eurasia and North America were now separate land masses, the evolutionary progress of the horse depended on developments within North America. Perhaps if *Hyracotherium* had still been about in Eurasia, things would have been different. As a rule if a branch is facing a dead end, a specialist population cannot revert to their ancestry and develop along new lines. With increased specialisation there is the opportunity for greater exploitation but there is also a greater dependence on the environment and a higher risk of extinction if things should change since the gene pool is initially more limited. Evolution does not allow second attempts or progress with the benefit of foresight. It simply builds on what is there.

Descendants of *Hyracotherium*

Within what was to become North America descendants arose who would ultimately replace *Hyracotherium*. These included the larger *Orohippus* and, later on, *Epihippus*. By the mid to late Oligocene, 35–25 million years ago, a more horse-like *Mesohippus* had appeared. *Mesohippus* probably lived in woodland close to swamps and at savannah–woodland borders. It had a more slender muzzle, more slender longer legs and was about 65 cm tall.

Mesohippus was the probable ancestor of *Miohippus*, and co-existed with *Miohippus* for about 5 million years. *Miohippus* was better adapted to the drier and more open regions including the expanding areas of grassland. Its teeth had more ridges and so were capable of breaking down a greater proportion of this tougher herbage. Even so *Miohippus* could still not survive by grazing alone.

Further climatic cooling and expansion of the grasslands during the Miocene epoch, which started around 22.5 million years ago and lasted till around 5 million years ago, provided another opportunity for adaptive radiation and migration of the genus. A large ice-cap developed over the South Pole and sea levels dropped as a result. Land appeared along the Bering Straits between North America and Siberia and horses were again able to migrate into Eurasia. Browsing species of horse continued to evolve in North America, but the appearance of truly grazing species of horse allowed the rapid recolonisation of the Eurasian continent and exploitation of the grasslands. Once again, the Old World hosted a family of horses and this time they were true grazers.

The grazers

These true grazing horses could exist because they had high crowned teeth which could resist the higher wear imposed by an all-grass diet. A similar feature happens to have arisen in cattle and sheep, which cope with the same problem. This phenomenon

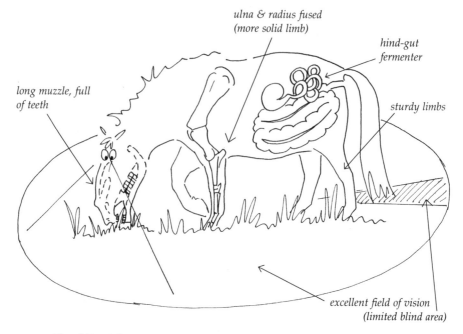

Fig. 3.5   Adaptations associated with an existence based on grasslands.

whereby the same trait arises in two or more species as a result of the same selective pressures is known as convergent evolution. It is not the result of a shared common ancestor. Other features of the grazing horses included the lateralisation of their eyes, which provides a wider field of view. The ability to detect predators from all sides and at a distance is undoubtedly important to horses living in more open grasslands and has important behavioural associations as we shall see in the next chapter. Predator pressure will soon favour those with a wider field of view.

Being big is an advantage when you are trying to avoid being eaten but the new open environment also appeared to favour certain survival behaviour strategies for horses, e.g. sustained flight in a straight line. Adaptation to this behaviour is not without its behavioural costs. A more efficient running stride occurs with the fusion of the lower limb bones to form a more solid limb. Set against this, though, is the reduced ability of the animal to turn sharply at speed. Horses are not adapted then to switching direction at speed but to sustaining their flight in one direction. Other grassland species adopt a different strategy for survival on the grasslands. Consider the small and nimble gazelle of Africa for example. This is games theory played out at the level of a whole ecosystem.

In the Old World, many of these new grazing horses had three toes and one group, *Hipparion*, survived until a few tens of thousands of years ago. A one-toed mutant arose in North America around 5 or 4 million years ago. This is known as *Pliohippus*, and this trait seems to have provided some form of advantage, as there soon radiated a whole family of similar individuals most notably *Dino-hippus*, the forerunner of *Equus*. This was about 1.4 metres at the withers and was stocky like a zebra. North and South America had joined together by this time and one toed grazers became the first horses in the southern sub-continent.

The arrival of Equus

There is considerable debate over the geographical origin of the modern horse genus *Equus*. The oldest recognisable fossils originate from the New World around 3 million years ago. Within 300 000 years, there is evidence of *Equus* in the South American, Eurasian and African continents. Migration would have been possible via the Bering land bridge, re-exposed by a northern glaciation which lowered the sea levels again about 2.5 million years ago. However, there are some differences between the teeth of zebras and the ancestors of the domestic horse.

One explanation would be that the genus arose from evolution in several places at about the same time and that there is no single ancestor for all modern horses. The technical way of saying this is that the horse has a polyphyletic origin as a result of parallel evolution. Parallel evolution is evolutionary change along similar lines as a result of similar but independent pressures on related, but reproductively isolated populations.

Opposing this view is evidence to suggest that the dental differences may not so much reflect a different ancestor, but a different environment, as a similar variation is seen in the large ruminants who are believed to share a common ancestor. This highlights the difficulty involved in interpreting fossil records and how the views of scientists are simply the best explanation of the available information. This is part of its attraction as there is so much room for progress by people who become fascinated by a particular aspect of the incomplete puzzle.

Today's wild horses
Today there are six recognised species of wild horse:

◇ **Three species of zebra** Some argue that the zebra's stripes are polyphyletic in origin and so zebras may not be as closely related as we think (see Bennett 1980).
◇ **Two species of ass** There are both an African and an Asian Ass. These have retained the ability to browse; a factor which has no

doubt been central to their survival. The Asian Ass is actually divided into two subspecies.

◇ **Przewalski's horse** This is the closest relative of the modern domestic horse. It is a true caballine horse like the domestic breeds, and probably the only real wild horse.

Other horses found in the wild are almost certainly feral populations, escaped from domestication.

From biochemical studies of the genetic components of cells and from fossil records, it would seem that the ancestors of the modern breeds of horse, *Equus caballus*, diverged from those of other modern day equids, like the zebra and the ass, about 1.5 million years ago.

Recent changes

Between 10 and 15000 years ago, the last ice age ended. This meant massive climatic and environmental change again. As the ice retreated, the Bering Sea separated North America and Asia and no further migration was possible. North America, the origin of the equids and their home for 55 million years, became a death-trap. The grasslands receded, being superseded by further extension of the woodlands, and the climate became more seasonal; so the availability of grazing fluctuated throughout the year. Obviously this was bad news for all the species that were specialised grazers. In fact 87% of the large mammalian species, including 40 genera, were wiped out. A further contributory factor to the horse's demise may have been the arrival of man as a hunter in the Americas at this time. Martin and Wright in their book on the Pleistocene extinctions suggest that the resident species were not adapted to this novel hunter, literally capable of 'overkill'. This may sound improbable, but a similar fate befell the horse's cousin the Quagga in South Africa in the nineteenth century. It took just a few decades for this species to go from enormous widespread free-ranging herds to extinction. The arrival of man is also often associated with more general non-specific environmental disruption, and this may indirectly affect the delicate ecosystem to which local animals have adapted. Whoever shoulders the blame, man or climatic change, the net result was that by 10000 years ago, all the equids had disappeared from North America.

Their relatives in the Old World faired slightly better. The global switch from extensive grasslands to more isolated grassland pockets resulted in the reproductive isolation of a number of populations. The situation was then set for these populations to evolve along their own independent lines.

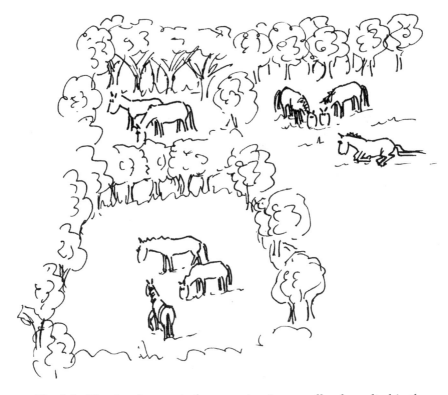

Fig. 3.6 The development of more extensive woodland resulted in the regional and reproductive isolation of a number of populations of horses.

The origins of the modern breeds

Since there were a number of discrete populations after the ice age it is generally agreed that there is no single line of descent for all the modern breeds. These are believed to have arisen from a number of populations or subspecies. Domestication may have occurred in one or a number of places and then spread around the globe with the migrants domesticating the local population.

Breed prototypes or vari-horse

The environment can mould subtle differences at a genetic level within a species. Evolution is not about the creation of species; it is about adaptation. So if there is variation within a species which can be acted on by natural selection, then we may see the development of regional characteristics. Thus regionally isolated populations in slightly different environments may be expected to vary when natural selection is allowed to operate. Whilst there are clear anatomical differences, there is little scientific knowledge about regional differences in behavioural tendency which may be associated with these. To illustrate this point we will show how a few physical and physiological limitations have come into play in different geographical areas, to produce subtly different populations.

Primitive Central European horse

This post-glacial population probably gave rise to many warm-blood types. A typical one was tall, standing at 1.7 m (15 hands), with fairly big feet, just the thing for running on soft grasslands without sinking too deep. It had a long, narrow skull with a slightly Roman nose and small piggy eyes. It also had a relatively large trunk. This means it had a low surface area to volume ratio, which tends to lead to less heat loss. Maintaining body temperature takes heat, which comes from food. This is an expensive way to use energy and so there is tremendous environmental pressure for adaptations to regulate heat loss in cooler climates. The observation that animals in lower environmental temperatures tend to have bigger trunks was first recorded by Bergman and is known as

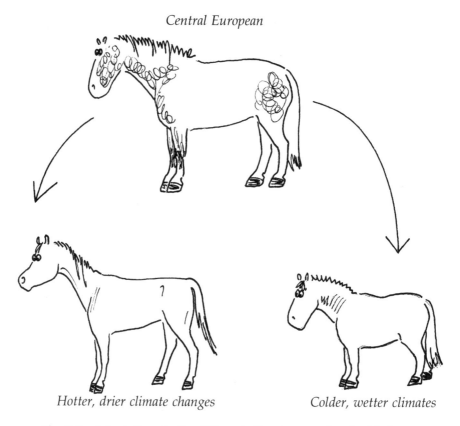

Central European

Hotter, drier climate changes   *Colder, wetter climates*

Fig. 3.7 Adaptations to the different climates associated with the Southern and Northern environments.

Bergman's Rule. A related observation has also been recorded and is known as Allen's Rule. This states that the extremities, like ears and legs, of animals tend to be smaller in those populations which have developed in colder climates. Both of these rules extend from the simple fact that spheres loose less heat from their surface than any other shape and heat conservation is important to warm-blooded animals in cold climates. The more you look like a sphere, the less heat you will lose relative to your volume.

Northern effects

Here the environment tends to be cooler, wetter and boggier. Accordingly we should not be surprised that the equine inhabitants of this region have large 'soup plate' feet, stubby limbs, a chunky body and short ears. They may also have a quite long Roman nose caused by an extended arching of the nasal bones (such as that which is typical of several Scandinavian and draft breeds). This is thought to allow the more effective warming of cold air before it passes down to the lungs. These features have been sought in many draft breeds.

Southern effects

Here daytime temperatures tend to be higher and the climate drier. Heat conservation is not so important but keeping cool is. Accordingly we may expect to see longer legs and ears, a lighter narrower trunk and a finer, shorter hair coat. As the climate is drier, the ground is harder and so there is no advantage to be gained from large feet. The drier air may favour the dishing of the face, so characteristic of breeds like the modern Arab. This is caused by the expansion of the bony cavities in the skull known as the frontal sinuses. It is believed that this helps moisten the air before it passes down to the lungs. Dry air in the lungs can result in serious damage from desiccation and reduces the efficiency of uptake of important gases like oxygen.

Domestication and its consequences

> Domestication is that process by which a population of animals becomes adapted to man and to the captive environment by some combination of genetic changes occurring over generations and environmentally induced developmental events reoccurring during each generation. (Price, 1984)

This suggests that the changes and differences we see between a wild and domestic animal may be the result of both genetic and developmental factors. If there is a problem with a domestic animal it is important to consider both of these possible origins for the condition in order to instigate appropriate treatment. But first let us consider what happens when we domesticate an animal and so how we can expect a domestic horse to differ from its wild relatives.

Selective breeding and culling

The process and consequences of domestication

When an animal is domesticated we usually ask (or force) it to live close to man and fit in with his lifestyle. In the early stages of domestication those that do not adapt are killed and so the population will change over time. We therefore see a form of evolution occurring in response to rules which differ from those in the wild. It is no longer a case of survival of the fittest, but survival of the most appropriate. Man has the power to interfere with breeding so mating is no longer random within the population but selective. Culling is also selective on certain traits and so if there is the potential for change in the population (i.e. the genes exist) then change may occur much more quickly in captivity.

Reduction of natural selection pressures

Man also cares for the domestic animal and so the pressure of natural selection on the efficiency of some behaviours is reduced. This includes behaviours ranging from parenting to eating, running away and normal social relations. Less fit animals and ones that would not otherwise live, survive because we look after them. This means we should not be surprised to see bad mothering or poor temperament persist in the population.

Intensification of the natural selection process

However, other aspects of natural selection are intensified largely because the domestic environment with its high population density can be very stressful for the individual. As a result:

(1) **There may be more aggression.** This is because individuals cannot get away from each other.
(2) **The risk of disease is intensified.** By living closer together it is easier for disease to spread from one individual to another.
(3) **Most behaviours become more relaxed.** This is because whilst stress can cause death it more often affects breeding performance and only those best adapted to this environment will survive to reproduce. These individuals are likely to be the generally less flighty and aggressive ones who conserve their energy for reproduction. Berger (1986) has also recorded how changes in social group structure tend to reduce reproductive performance.

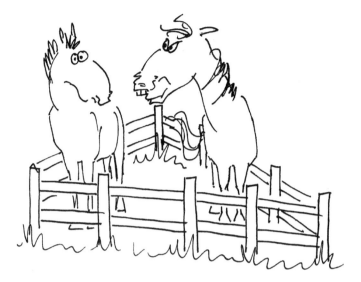

Fig. 3.8 Confinement can lead to intensification of any aggression.

(4) **Sexual behaviour can be expected to intensify.** The artificially large group sizes in which most domestic animals are kept means that the most precocious and promiscuous of those allowed to breed will tend to breed more and extend these traits through the generations. Feist (1971) reports distinct mare colour preferences within the harems of feral stallions. This tends not to be tolerated or allowed in the domestic situation, where males are expected to be less fussy about their sexual partners, but it may still arise occasionally. Such selectivity and poor reproductive performance may be identified as a specific breeding problem when it is really a natural phenomenon associated with the environment and the individual.

(5) **Recessive homozygosity can occur.** This is an apparent increase in the appearance of traits that are normally masked by more dominant genes. This is because captive populations tend to be more closed than wild ones and so there is an increased tendency to inbreeding. Sometimes these states are fatal at an early stage of foetal development and so nothing is born but at other times they have a quite stunning appearance, e.g. albinism, or the hair type which gives rise to the characteristic mane of the Norwegian Fjord pony, or the gait of the Missouri Foxtrotter. Once a curious feature such as this arises it may be selectively bred for in order to spread it through a population. Thus features which would either rarely or never be seen in a wild population come to be a common feature of a domestic one and may even form the basis of a breed standard.

Modern breeds therefore largely reflect the physiological adaptations that occur in response to a stressful environment and man's curious fascination with the preservation of the unusual whenever it occurs. Only in more recent (post-Renaissance) times have specific breeding strategies been undertaken to develop horses for specific purposes such as racing or to meet a particular breed standard.

Neotenisation

It has been suggested that domestication results in the persistence of juvenile features within the individual at both the physical and behavioural level. A change known as neotenisation. There are several possible explanations as to why this may have occurred.

(1)   Firstly, it is suggested that the behaviour of young animals is more flexible than that of adults and so more desirable and likely to be selected for in captivity.

(2)   Alternatively these behaviours may persist into adulthood because the pressure for the development of more mature behaviours (with the exception of sexual behaviour) has been reduced through the protection afforded by the captive environment.

(3)   Alternatively, the juvenile behaviours may persist because they have been rewarded and so the animals have been conditioned by man during development to continue to behave in this way (see Chapter 9). In effect they have never been psychologically weaned or forced to grow up.

(4)   Other possible explanations suggest that biological and/or physical characteristics within the environment inhibit the development of adult behaviour patterns. For example, animals reared in same-age groups will be isolated from adults and as a result may never learn normal adult behaviour.

It is very difficult to demonstrate which, if any, of these factors are relevant or how comparatively important they may be, although such information would help us to improve our management of horses in the long run.

The taming of the horse

Since the wild and domestic horse differ little in archaeological appearance it is difficult to establish when the horse was first tamed. This certainly happened after domestication of the dog, sheep, goat and cow and may reflect the general unsuitability or poor adaptability of the horse to the domestic environment. This is in contrast to its close relative the ass which was successfully domesticated in Africa some time before the horse. As a larger, more agile animal with quite specific dietary requirements and a tendency to migrate over large distances, it would have taken a lot of skill and effort for Stone Age man to keep and look after a captive horse.

The abundant distribution of chopped horse bones amidst signs of human settlement around Dereivka, between the Black and Caspian Seas, would seem to suggest that horses started their domestic life as a feature of the neolithic menu about five thousand years ago. In this region it seems that man stalked horses, whereas further east in Botai, Kazakhstan, he seems to have hunted them by driving them off cliffs or into swamps. At this time cattle were already being used for draught purposes, but the potential of the horse as a beast of burden was soon realised. Where this was done first we do not know, but the power of the horse combined with the development of the spoked chariot wheel extended man's conquering abilities.

The art of riding and horsemanship developed thereafter within about 500 years. This enabled invaders from Asia, possibly following drought in their native land, to cross more easily over the wooded and marshland areas that covered Europe at that time (about 1700 BC). Settlers arrived in Egypt and India about 100 years later. The immigrants would have bred their horses with those available locally and spread the skill of domestication and equitation.

The horse has never competed well with man and become extinct in the wild wherever there has been a high density of human inhabitants. It is therefore somewhat ironic that its domestication, by extending man's mobility, probably hastened its initial extinction in the wild but secured its survival as a species both in the domestic and non-captive state. Those caballine horses which exist in the wild today, with the possible exception of the Przewalski horse, are not wild untamed ancestors but more probably reintroduced populations or feral escapees from the domestic situation. Some, like the Exmoor, have probably been wild for hundreds of generations and have developed their own breed standard through natural selection. More recently feral populations like the mustang do not breed so true.

Evolution into mythology

A few interesting footnotes were probably left in mythology by this spread of the horse. Firstly the extensive use of the horse by the Scythians to the north east of Greece probably represents the origin of stories relating to the Centaurs. As the first Greek riders did not appear until some time later, these able horseman must have appeared like an alien creature, half man half beast. The accounts of sea-gods like the Greek Poseidon, with a chariot pulled by horses over the water, may also reflect how domestic horses first arrived in some islands, i.e. on ships across the sea.

TOPICS FOR DISCUSSION

◇ What traits in an animal would make its domestication easier?
◇ What aspects of domestic horse management is the horse likely to be adapted to as a result of previous selective processes? Are these traits of the pre- or post-domestication period?
◇ What aspects of domestic horse management is the horse unlikely to be adapted to as a result of previous selection?
◇ Domestication does not produce qualitative changes in behaviour, just quantitative changes. Discuss.
◇ Is the horse a supreme athlete or the best available model of an old design?
◇ What does it mean to be a horse?
◇ How might horses change if they were isolated for 10 million years on an island, without man or predators and subject to global warming by 15 degrees? Consider the conditions that apply to your proposed adaptation.

References and further reading

Bennett, D.K. (1980) Stripes do not a zebra make. Part I. A cladistic analysis of *Equus. Systematic Zoology* **29**, 272–87.

Berger, J. (1986) *Wild Horses of the Great Basin*. University of Chicago Press, Chicago.

Clutton-Brock, J. (1987) *A Natural History of Domesticated Mammals*. Cambridge University Press, Cambridge.

Clutton-Brock, J. (1992) *Horse Power*. Natural History Museum Publications, London.

Feist, F.D. (1971) *Behavior of feral horses in the Pryor Mountain Wild Horse Range*. MSc Thesis, University of Michigan.

Hemmer, H. (1990) *Domestication, the Decline of Environmental Appreciation*. Cambridge University Press, Cambridge.

MacFadden, B.J. (1992) *Fossil Horses: Systematics, Palaeobiology and Evolution of the Family Equidae*. Cambridge University Press, Cambridge.

Martin, P.S. & Wright, H.E. (1967) *Pleistocene Extinctions: the Search for a Cause*. Yale University Press, New Haven.

Price, E.O. (1984) Behavioral aspects of domestication. *The Quarterly Review of Biology* **55** (1), 1–32.

4. The Lifetime Development of Behaviour

So far we have considered how equine behaviour has developed through evolution. In this chapter we examine the development of behaviour during the lifetime of an individual. This builds on the genetic foundation provided by evolution but allows some manipulation within the domestic situation.

Instinctive and learned behaviour, what is the difference?

When considering the development (or ontogeny) of behaviour we must remember that both normal and problem behaviour development is the result of the continuous interaction of genetic and environmental factors (see Chapter 2). The genetic code is fixed at conception and cannot be changed. The genetic blueprint will therefore apply certain restrictions on what is and what is not practicable, but an animal will not develop appropriately without the right cues from the environment. Thus nature and nurture are inseparable.

Nonetheless we still refer to instinctive behaviour patterns; so what do we mean if they are not genetically determined? The types of behaviour that we tend to refer to as instinctive, such as suckling, standing, running and neighing, tend to be nearly complete the first time they are expressed although they are still fine-tuned and modified by learning. The association between the behaviour and the consequence also tends to be made very rapidly, after perhaps a single short exposure. For example, the foal's first fumbling attempts at suckling may soon gain it some milk, but there is room for some improvement with experience once the association between teat and milk has been made.

Learned behaviours take much longer to develop and are much more obviously affected by the environment. For example, an unhandled youngster will not automatically pick his foot up for you the first time you ask, but he soon learns the routine once it has been repeated several times. There has not been any change in the biological ability of either the suckling foal or the unhandled youngster. In both of these circumstances the horse has simply become more efficient at doing something it was physically capable of doing all along. The differentiation between an instinctive and a learned behaviour would seem to be determined by how much learning the animal has to do, and as some behaviours come more easily to the naive animal than others, the definitions of learned and instinctive behaviour are relative.

Instinctive behaviours tend to be triggered by fairly general events or impressions, known as sign stimuli. Most of the 'hardware' required for their expression is already loosely linked together at birth. This also means that they are less open to modification by the environment, a property which has earned them the title of 'fixed action patterns', or 'fixed motor patterns'. If the environment in which the animal lives is different to that in which the behaviour pattern evolved the animal may display a totally inappropriate behaviour and be labelled 'stupid'. This is not the case. Like all aspects of behaviour that fit within an evolutionary framework, it is well adapted for the function it was intended to perform. Imagine what would happen if a foal had to learn exactly how to suckle from scratch. It would be dead before it had its first drink. Instinctive behaviour patterns tend to be seen in situations where the required response is vital to immediate survival. In situations such as these, behavioural flexibility is not a priority.

The great advantage of learning is that it increases an animal's flexibility and the ability to adapt within one lifetime.

Building complex behaviours from more simple ones

Problems arise with instinctive behaviours when the animal responds to the wrong cues. This most often happens because of unintentional cues for the behaviour in the domestic environment. Take for example the first suckling of the newborn foal. Fraser (1992) suggests that in order to do this a foal must complete successfully a number of stages of behavioural development:

(1) **Recumbent co-ordination** – getting itself together on the floor
(2) **Rising and quadrupedal stability** – standing
(3) **Ambulation** – walking
(4) **Maternal orientation** – identifying the right thing to head for
(5) **Teat-seeking and sucking** – drinking.

The smells and noises associated with the release of milk then help the foal to identify the goal more specifically in future. There is therefore a lot of learning involved in even this basic task. Once the foal has started to suckle, the actual pattern and style of the

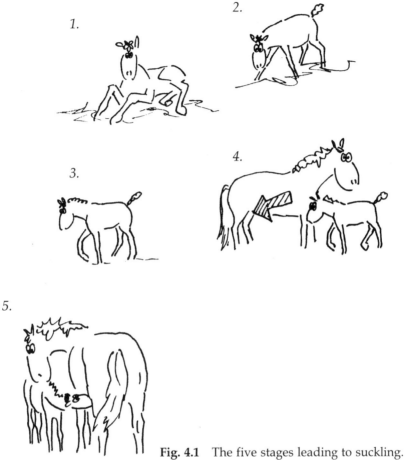

Fig. 4.1   The five stages leading to suckling.

behaviour become modified as the foal learns the most efficient way of obtaining milk from the teat.

The foal is not born with a picture of its mother and the knowledge of what she can provide inside its head, but it may be born with a behavioural tendency to head towards a dark undersurface. In the wild, the mare will often be separate from the rest of the herd when she foals and stands before her foal. It is very likely, therefore, that the only dark undersurface in the area will be her belly. The programme the foal has is sufficient and efficient for its purpose in these circumstances but in other circumstances there is a risk that the programme will not prove as effective. The foal will head towards the nearest dark area, which may be a fixed manger in the corner of the stable or an interfering human. The flexibility of instinctive behaviours is very limited.

However once the task has been performed with some degree of effective feedback the response becomes less open and more

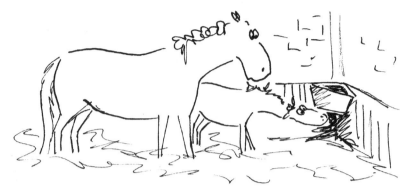

Fig. 4.2   Sometimes instinctive behaviour patterns can go wrong.

specific. As a result, these bouts of important behaviour development and learning have been called 'critical periods' or 'sensitive
phases'.

Sensitive phases for special times and specific associations

Since the term 'critical period' was first used, we have learnt that
these periods are not as critical as first thought. The timing is not
quite as fixed and the establishment of the behaviour not quite so
rigid, and so currently behaviour scientists prefer to describe them
as 'sensitive phases'. The main feature of these life stages is that they
represent a time when the animal is particularly susceptible to
certain learning experiences.

The neonatal phase

This is characterised by the foal learning to stand, walk and nurse
and results in primary socialisation.

The phase lasts only about two hours or up to the point at which
the first milk is drunk. It involves the identification of a leading
mother and other close companions. A tolerance or even affection
develops for anything which does not disturb the foal or its mother
figure at this time. Introducing people now who do not upset the
mare will help establish a strong human–foal bond and ease later
training. This factor is exploited in the 'imprint training' technique
promoted by Robert Miller (1991) and explained in more detail
below.

The transitional phase

This lasts about two weeks. It is called the transitional phase as it
represents the time of greatest sensory development.

Again biases may occur as a result of experiences at this time. It is suspected that foals with very little sensory exposure at this time have a reduced sensory capacity. As a result they may be less able to discriminate subtle differences and appear clumsy or easily spooked. However, excessive stimulation may also be detrimental as it may lay the foundation for a restless individual who constantly seeks activity A similar principle probably underlies the development of certain aspects of the emotions around this time. More work is needed in this area in order for us to develop rearing systems that maximise the mental robustness of horses and their ability to cope with the rigors of the domestic environment. During the transitional phase the foal remains close to its mother and probably learns behaviour strategies from her responses to the environment as well as its own experiences.

The socialisation phase

As social play peaks at around four weeks, the foal enters the socialisation phase. Other aspects of play also peak during this time, which extends until the foal is about 12 weeks of age. Such aspects include the expression of behaviours like jaw snapping and mutual grooming. Snapping tends to occur when a young animal makes an initial approach to another larger one and is occasionally directed towards non-equids. The behaviour may be more common when there is some uncertainty about the outcome of the approach, i.e. whether the response will be friendly or hostile. It is important to recognise and distinguish jaw snapping from a bite threat. In jaw snapping the lips are pulled back to expose a set of champing teeth, with a bite threat the ears are laid back and the lips retracted as the neck is stretched forward.

The juvenile phase

During this phase, play and other activities are focused on the development of adult social skills which will affect the horse's ultimate position in the herd. After this the horse enters puberty and becomes a fully mature adult.

The maturation of behaviour

The physical development of the horse may accompany the appearance of behaviour patterns associated with a particular stage of life. For example, the development of sexual behaviour depends first on the development of the hormone secreting glands which control it.

This process is known as behavioural maturation and it is another form of behaviour development. The animal does not necessarily have to learn what is required, but it does have to wait until the nerves responsible for expressing and co-ordinating the behaviour have developed. During sensitive phases it may be that the pathways associated with certain links in the brain are just ripe for connecting and the experiences of the young animal at this time lead to specific links being made. In the neonatal phase, the source of the first reward to the foal may lead it to use that object as a guide and model for its actions. This can cause problems as Konrad Lorenz found with his geese (Lorenz, 1961). When geese hatch they follow and imprint on whatever they see first. This phenomenon is quite common in many birds and is similar to the bonding of a foal to its mother after the first feed. Lorenz was responsible for leading these birds to water for the first time, and found that they would not enter until he first took the plunge. This effect is long lasting and not easy to overcome even by exposure to the right biological role model. When the birds matured, this caused particular problems as some displayed their affections towards Lorenz rather than the other geese. A similar problem has occasionally been reported in pet miniature ponies which are taken in and brought up with a human family.

Using play for better management

Solitary and social play

Many of the behaviours, which are required later in life appear in what looks like a practice form or play first. It may involve interaction with others (social play) or be solitary. Solitary play, such as skipping around or manipulating object, and play with the mother, such as nibbling and nipping, tend to be quite frequent soon after birth and fall steadily over the next few months. At the same time social play with other horses tends to increase. Young animals, in particular, appear to spend large amounts of time and energy playing; for example, young colts will often mount things before they are sexually mature. From an evolutionary point of view this would tend to indicate that it is very important to the individual. However it may almost totally disappear when times are hard. So whilst being important to the individual it is not essential to life.

Natural benefits of play

In people play is believed to be essential for the development of normal healthy adult behaviour and a similar argument could be put forward for its role in animals even though the available evidence from other species suggests that practice and play are not crucial in this way. It may be that play helps to refine an individual's skill or shape certain behavioural tendencies. So colts reared in groups become more efficient at mounting. It may also be at this time that individual preferences start to develop.

Time spent in play is also time spent learning and exercising so the playful individual may be fitter and more aware of its physical and social environments. This means it can develop behaviour strategies and tactics which may be of importance later in life. If you want a sure-footed horse you should let it wander on a regular basis over as many uneven surfaces as you can find. Play fights and conflicts help indicate an individual's strengths and weaknesses without risk of injury and may suggest its later position within the herd as a mature adult.

Whilst it is actually quite difficult to say whether or not a certain activity is a playful one, unless it is preceded by an obvious signal such as a small nip, play is only really recognised in species of animal with an emotional brain (that is, with the 'hardware' necessary to feel pleasure and to suffer). It also appears to occur most readily in animals whose vital needs for survival have been met and starts either spontaneously from within an individual or following encouragement and invitation from another. These observations would tend logically to suggest that true play is a pleasurable experience and so good for a horse's well-being. Play is a very useful and beneficial way of filling time when it is available. It may therefore have a lot of use in the management of the stabled horse as we shall see later in Chapter 10.

Making play out of work

Fraser (1992) suggests that we should try to make play out of the work we require from a horse. It may be that if we teach a horse to play chase (or even better to play the lead of a chase) we may have a horse that enjoys running and is an efficient runner. This makes for happy and probably more successful racehorses. Similar ideas could be developed for other equitation disciplines. It is also easier to control a horse which wants to please rather than one which is afraid to disobey as we shall see when we discuss the effects of punishment (see Chapter 9). This idea produces winners all around and so is worthy of careful consideration in the development of any horse's training programme.

Successful and purposive play

Emotional tendencies, like behavioural tendencies, are probably largely established early in life. The experiences of the foal are therefore likely to be very important in developing his temperament. Confidence comes from being successful in a wide variety of situations and so it is important that we give the foal many opportunities to be successful in its play. Play should be fun but focus on the purpose for which we want the horse.

This knowledge can be applied to improve the management of domestic horses through the development of training programmes, which match your needs with those of your horse and its natural behavioural development.

Using natural biases in development to improve management

Optimal behaviour development is about encouraging the development of the right skills at the right time. In the wild this often happens as a result of sensitive learning phases and interaction with certain horses at appropriate ages; in the domestic situation most horses are deprived of some of this opportunity to interact and learn from others. In this case it is our responsibility to take on this role. The domestic situation also makes different demands on the horse, for example with regards to work. It is therefore useful to design exercises to prepare the horse for a domestic rather than wild existence and so make domestic life less stressful. The exercises should help to ensure the development of a confident and well-mannered horse with the fundamental skills which it will require later in life. Specific programmes can be developed to meet your personal requirements but they should always be applied with a full awareness of the principles of learning described later in Chapter 9.

In considering imprint training and maturation training below we outline some general exercises which can easily be adapted to meet your own requirements.

Imprint training

The technique described here is based on that of Robert Miller (1991). Further details on the method can be found in his book, details of which are given at the end of the chapter. The term 'imprint' may be somewhat misleading, as the process does not involve imprinting in the normal sense of the word. Imprint training is designed to teach the foal to tolerate and accept future experiences which it may otherwise find aversive. This is done by exposing the new-born horse to a variety of stimuli until they are tolerated without resistance.

Advantages of the technique

This has several advantages. Firstly it is physically easier to handle and manipulate a young foal and so establish tolerance of being handled and restrained. Secondly, the desired behavioural strategy is established in the young animal before it has learned any alternative and so there is no resistance from other reinforced strategies. The new behaviour should therefore be easier to establish.

Effects of the technique
So long as there is no need for the horse to behave otherwise, the animal can be expected to continue to behave in the learned way, i.e. the behaviour is likely to persist as long as the learned response is appropriate and effective. Controlled exposure and elimination of any fear response at this age has a lasting effect as the brain has a tendency to use the strategies which worked the first time in future situations. This helps to explain why it is usually easier to train consistent behaviour patterns in younger animals.

Timing of the procedures
Training can be started soon after the mare has stood following the birth of the foal. She should however be allowed to lick and smell the foal first. Care must be taken not to upset the mare at this time as she may react aggressively to the intrusion. The mare is haltered and allowed contact with the foal throughout the exercises. As a rule of thumb, the foal is handled or the procedure repeated at least until it relaxes. This way the foal learns to habituate properly to the stimulus (see Chapter 9). The first group of exercises may be performed before the foal even stands. They include the following:

(1) **The face and head** are handled all over, including inside the ears, mouth and nostrils. This latter procedure will ease the acceptance of a stomach tube later in life.
(2) **The trunk and limbs** are rubbed except around the lower flank where the leg aid is applied, an area that should be left sensitive to touch. Particular attention should be paid to the perineal area so that it is never difficult to take the animal's temperature.
(3) **The soles of the feet** are firmly but gently tapped with the palm of the hand in order to ensure tolerance of farriery procedures.

This is likely to take at least an hour and the foal should be restrained throughout.

Desensitisation
After the foal has suckled, he can be desensitised to a wider range of environmental stimuli over the first few days. Again it is important to keep the foal restrained so that each procedure can be continued until it is completely accepted. This should reduce the risk of spooking. Key tests include:

(1)   Exposure to the sound and vibration of clippers.
(2)   Being rubbed with plastic sheeting. This is noisy and produces an unusual sensation, habituating the foal to a range of novelties.
(3)   The sound of traffic and other machinery. This should be done on a private road where it can all be safely stage managed. It is best to start with smaller and slower machinery like lawn mowers and to introduce larger vehicles in later exercises. Tape recordings may be used to add further distractions and stimulation to an otherwise quiet road.
(4)   The sound of clattering dustbin lids.
(5)   The application of leg bandages. The desensitisation of the legs earlier should make this task easy.
(6)   The pressure of a surcingle.
(7)   Pressure over the saddle area. This should be applied with the palms of the hands.
(8)   Straddling the foal without applying pressure to its back.
(9)   The feel of blankets.
(10) The sight, sound and feel of loose plastic bags strapped around its body. In this exercise the foal does not need to be restrained so long as it cannot dislodge the bags. The more it moves the greater the novelty of stimulation and effectiveness of the exercise. The bags must not be removed until the foal is completely calm with them on.
(11) The feel of a head-collar and being tied up. It is essential that the mother is kept nearby at this time.
(12) Tolerance of feet being picked up and held.

Initiating a response
Around the same time it is worth sensitising the foal to respond appropriately to the slightest touch in certain areas. In this procedure, the pressure should stop as soon as he moves in the right direction. The object here is to establish a learned association as early as possible. The foal will then learn the appropriate response through negative reinforcement (see Chapter 9). Again this is easier in younger animals for the reasons given above.

(1)   Gentle pressure behind the rump to move him forward.
(2)   Gentle pressure on the chest to move him back.
(3)   Gentle pressure to the flanks to move him over.
(4)   The use of a halter to lead him in any direction.

If the foal is stood perpendicular to and in front of the mare, the halter should be pulled gently towards the mare. It is then more likely that the foal will actually step towards its mother rather than just turn its head towards her. Any steps in the right direction should be rewarded by the release of pressure from the halter. A foal can be taught to lead on the halter in a similar way. He is stood alongside his mother and as he is moved forward a second handler leads the mare on. His natural following response will encourage and reward the appropriate behaviour. With a bit of patience the foal will soon lead in hand perfectly.

These exercises should all be started in the first week and perhaps once or twice more in the next week. They will then need only occasional reinforcement later.

Maturation training

Another group of exercises, which should also be started early in the foal's life, relate to the development of its brain and body for safe, co-ordinated riding later in life. We call this 'maturation training'. The development and refinement of these skills is more dependent on exposure over a longer period of time and extends through the transitional and socialisation phases. However, there is no need to wait until the horse is a few years old before you prepare him for riding. Even though the horse is not being ridden, if left untrained he could be establishing certain behavioural tendencies which might interfere with the riding process. We need to set him up to fulfil his potential from the start rather than try to iron out the wrinkles that have developed in his lifetime. In order to undertake these exercises effectively and safely it is important to make sure first that you can easily lead the horse in hand.

(1)   **Sure-footedness** The foal should be walked over a variety of uneven and slightly unsure surfaces on a regular basis. This will encourage co-ordination and sure-footedness.

(2)   **Horse boxes** The foal should be led into a horse box and allowed to feed. It should not be transported the first time, nor allowed to leave until it appears perfectly calm. Ideally a variety of boxes and lorries should be used on a number of occasions. This should help avoid loading problems later in life. If access to a trailer is not possible then sheets of metal could be used to build suitable ramps as a substitute, since it seems that one of the most aversive aspects of loading is the sensation produced from walking on a hollow surface.

(3)   **Light and shade** The foal should be required to move from light areas into darker ones in order to suckle from its mother on a number of occasions. Many herbivores have a tendency to avoid entering a dark building or cross light–dark boundaries, for example at barn entrances, because they cannot see very clearly when the light suddenly changes. This exercise should be practised during the first two weeks, when sensory development is at its peak.

(4)   **Loads** Light packs should be applied to the back of the foal so that it builds up the necessary back support which will reduce the risk of degeneration later in life. As a rule of thumb no more than 15% of the foal's body weight should be used. This exercise should continue until the foal is properly backed, the weight being gradually increased in preparation for a rider.

(5)   **Weaning** This is an inevitably distressing time for both mares and foals. It may also be the time when a number of stereotypic behaviour problems are established (see Chapter 10). It may be possible to reduce the stress of weaning by getting the foal used to being alone and away from its mother for ever increasing periods of time beforehand. Group weaning is preferable to box weaning and the foals should be encouraged to play with each other at this time. Alternatively they could be provided with some distraction, for example toys to play with, in order to prevent them engaging in repetitive behaviours such as fence or box walking and cross-suckling.

(6)   **Response to signals** Loose schooling to teach the appropriate response to voice and body signals should begin before the foal is a year old. For this a 10–15 metre round pen or circular area enclosed by jumps is most useful. Loose schooling should be followed by long-reining rather than lungeing as the foal is not yet skeletally mature and persistent circling may lead to problems later. As your horse learns how to respond to various commands, it is worth slowly introducing distractions as you reinforce these exercises. These should be sufficiently distracting for him to show the slightest sign of interest, such as an occasionally cocked ear, but should not interfere with his performance. With time you will find that his ability to concentrate on the task in hand improves and he is not deterred by ever more disturbing stimuli.

(7)   **Posture** It is also easier to work on building the ideal move-ment posture at this age in order to prevent the problems associated with a sunken back. Pole work will encourage him to look down and raise his back as a result.

(8)   **Problem solving skills and learning flexibility** These can be encouraged by the provision of a rich and varied environment. Problem tasks may also be set in a free school situation. For example the foal may be required to negotiate a small maze in order to gain access to a special feed. Another simple task is to separate the foal from a reward by a length of fencing with a gap at one or both ends. The foal then has to learn to go round to get the food. This teaches it that the direct route is not the only possibility. If necessary the foal can be led through the solution until it gets the idea. These tricks take advantage of a horse's strong tendency to explore on its own, which can be seen in wild horses from the age of about one year.

(8)   **Social interactions** The foal should also be given the opportunity to learn the common language of horses. This is done best by
allowing him to mix freely with other horses of all ages. It is
important that these role models are familiar with foals in order to
avoid unnecessary injury. They will then teach him the subtle language of threat and submission by which physical contact and
injury in groups of horses are usually avoided.

These exercises prepare the horse both mentally and physically for
the rigours of domestic life. An early investment in managing the
behaviour of the foal soon pays dividends. If good behaviour is
taught from the outset, bad habits do not have to be eliminated
before effective training can begin because they have never been
learned.

Conclusion

The domestic horse is not the same as the wild one and we must be
cautious about the comparisons we make between the two. Both are
subjected to pressures which encourage the development of traits
which are adaptive to survival in the given environment. The rate of
change in captivity is potentially much greater than anything in the
wild to which the horse population over many generations or an
individual horse in its own lifetime could adapt. The horse is only
fully able to cope if the necessary genes exist in the population or if
its brain and behaviour are flexible enough to allow development
within the lifetime of the individual. Later we will see what sort of
adaptation the horse is likely to be capable of, so we can honestly
assess where the breed and the individual may have problems in
captivity. Part Two looks at how nature has equipped the horse for
living and Part Three looks further into how flexible an individual's
behaviour may be in unnatural situations.

TOPICS FOR DISCUSSION

◇ It has been suggested that behaviour develops through 'natural
selection' of appropriate brain connections. Consider the implications of this idea for training and retraining horses.
◇ Consider how and at what age you could encourage the expression
of suitable traits in a foal bred for dressage or racing.
◇ How might we prepare a foal for some of the stresses associated
with a life in captivity?
◇ Imprinting is the rapid learning of certain behaviours during
sensitive phases. The learning is then very stable if not irreversible.
How does this compare to 'imprint training'?

References and further reading

Boy, V. & Duncan, P. (1979) Time budgets of Camargue horses. Part I. Developmental changes in the time budgets of foals. *Behaviour* **71**, 187–202.

Brownlee, A. (1984) Animal play. *Applied Animal Behaviour Science* **12**, 307–312.

Fagan, R. (1981) *Animal Play Behaviour*. Oxford University Press, Oxford.

Fraser, A.F. (1989) Horse play as an ethosystem. *Etologia* **1**, 9–17.

Fraser, A.F. (1992) *The Behaviour of the Horse*. CAB International, Wallingford.

Lorenz, K. (1961) *King Solomon's Ring*. Methuen & Co., Cambridge.

Miller, R.M. (1991) *Imprint Training of the New-born Foal*. Western Horseman Inc., Colorado Springs.

Rees, L., (1993) *The Horse's Mind*. Stanley Paul. London.

Part 2
Mechanisms of Behaviour

In this section we consider the nuts and bolts of behaviour. The anatomy and physiology of behaviour determine its biases and flexibility. It is important to understand this aspect in order to appreciate its complexity and how different a horse's mind is likely to be from our own. Here we have clear physical evidence of differences not just a theoretical argument. We need to appreciate this level of behavioural origin, since it is only with this knowledge that we can really understand the implications of most physical interventions on behaviour, whether they be drugs, nutrient supplements or surgical procedures. In the second part of this section we examine some of the characteristic behaviour patterns of horses, why these have arisen and how the domestic situation is likely to effect them. From this we can devise techniques for more effective management.

5. The Processing of Information

Introduction

Horses receive stimuli constantly from both their internal and external environment. These stimuli provide the horse with information it needs, not only to stay alive but also to stay healthy. Stimuli provide information which may be acted on by the nervous system, the endocrine system, or both. The nervous and endocrine systems are the two major control systems in the body. Most mechanisms contributing to maintenance of the body have neural and endocrine components. Co-ordination of the two usually occurs at the level of the hypothalamus in the brain. Nervous responses to stimuli tend to be faster than endocrine responses. However the endocrine system should not be thought of as being 'slow'; many of its functions are carried out within seconds although others take days. The nervous system is considered in some detail below and aspects of the endocrine system are discussed in Chapter 8 on the sexual and reproductive behaviour of horses and in the section on stress in Chapter 10.

The nervous system

Fundamental features

The nervous system is like an electrical circuit board, it has inputs and outputs, with various means of data processing in between. Whilst we have not unravelled the entire circuit board, we know a great deal about how it works, and how simple 'programmes' for nervous function can be written. The nervous system has three basic components:

(1) **Sensory system (input)** The receptor cells and sense organs.
(2) **Central nervous system (data processing)** The brain and spinal cord.
(3) **Motor system (output)** Consisting of the autonomic and somatic motor systems.

Stimuli

A stimulus can be thought of as a trigger for a nerve impulse. The stimulus can be chemical, mechanical, photic or electrical and can arise internally or externally. An example of an external mechanical stimulus is the pressure of your leg against the horse's skin. Stimuli are detected by specialised receptor cells, which are designed to respond to a particular type of stimulus. The stimulus can be thought of as the input to the nervous system; it gives information or raw data regarding the internal and external environment. The stimuli that the horse receives are no different to those that you or I respond to, but the way in which they are detected, processed and responded to determine the differences in our behaviour.

Processing information

All stimuli, regardless of format, are converted to electrical signals which pass along the membranes of nerves. Electrical circuits are built from three components:

(1) **Sensory neurones** These carry information from the receptors to the central nervous system and make up the afferent nervous system.
(2) **Motor neurones** These carry information from the central nervous system to the organs which are responsible for bringing about a change. Those nerves that go to the muscles for locomotion and movement make up the somatic motor system, whilst those which go to the organs and viscera of the body make up the autonomic nervous system.
(3) **Inter-neurones** These make up most of the central nervous system and are responsible for co-ordinating the various inputs and outputs so that a coherent response is made.

One of the simplest electrical circuits is that of a sensory nerve, a connecting inter-neurone within the grey matter of the spinal cord and a motor neurone in series. Circuits like this produce reflex actions, like the knee jerk. More complex behaviours may depend on the integration of millions or billions of neurones.

If animals are to bring about highly specific motor actions or behaviour patterns in response to stimuli, the trafficking of electrical information throughout the nervous system must be tightly controlled. This is achieved through the use of chemical synapses between nerves. Chemical signals known as neurotransmitters are used to translate the electrical information across the gap between cells known as a synapse. There are few places within the body where direct electrical connection is used to transmit nerve impulses from one nerve to another. Chemical transmission of impulses across synapses is essential in the coding of neural information and

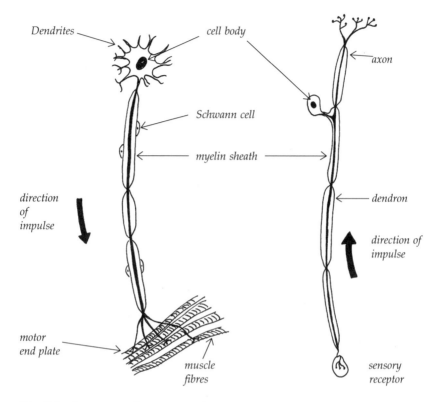

Fig. 5.1   Structure of sensory and motor neurones.

provides an opportunity for the modification of behaviour through the use of drugs and other chemicals.

Receptors

Receptors are found externally and internally, and it is these that determine the nature of the sensation not the stimulus. Receptors are most sensitive to the type of stimulus to which they are designed to respond, and are less sensitive, yet not insensitive to others. For example, the photoreceptors of the eye are designed to respond to light, yet if pressure is put on the eyeball, light is seen; the receptors are activated even though it was not the appropriate stimulus. Receptors can be simply the nerve endings of sensory neurones. Modified (e.g. encapsulated) nerve endings, form the basis of more complex receptors, whilst others are separate cells, or groups of cells. The over-stimulation of almost any receptor is perceived centrally as painful. For example very bright lights can hurt although they do not stimulate any pain fibres directly.

The 'catchment area' of a receptor, i.e. the region in which the application of an appropriate stimulus results in a nerve impulse

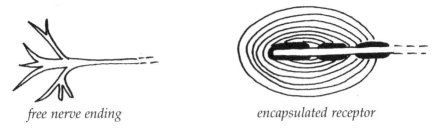

free nerve ending   encapsulated receptor

Fig. 5.2   Types of simple sensory receptor.

being initiated within the receptor, is known as the 'receptive field'. Small receptive fields produce high discrimination, i.e. a good ability to distinguish between two separate but similar stimuli, whilst large receptive fields lead to low discrimination.

The types and power of receptors varies between species and we must try to appreciate the world through a horse's senses if we wish to understand its behaviour. Horses are more sensitive to movement and certain sounds than humans; they also have a wider field of vision but are not as able to discriminate fine detail. So they will detect and respond to a different range of stimuli in the same environment compared to us. It is important to appreciate this before we jump to conclusions about why a horse is behaving in a certain way. The sensory capacity of individuals also varies as a result of development, with the special senses being particularly sensitive to environmental factors during the transitional phases (see Chapter 4).

Neural transmission

The transmission of impulses around the nervous system forms the framework on which behaviour is built. An understanding of the processes forms the basis of a mechanistic explanation of behaviour.

The initial stimulus causes a change in the electrical charge across the cell membrane. This process is known as 'depolarisation' and the result is known as a 'generator potential'. In order for the stimulus to be registered, it must cause depolarisation of the nerve membrane beyond a set point for that nerve. This set point is known as the 'threshold potential'. Provided the generator potential is greater than the threshold potential, a nerve impulse will be fired. Usually, the stronger the stimulus, the greater the generator potential. Nerve impulses are carried by series of action potentials; these are carried like a wave of negative electrical charge along the outside of the nerve fibre. The greater the generator potential, the greater the frequency of action potentials along the nerve.

Action potentials

Nerves and muscle fibres are both capable of transmitting action potentials. Together they are known as 'excitable tissue'. The distribution of ions across the membrane is such that the inside of the membrane is at about −70 milliVolts relative to the outside. Depolarisation causes the opening of voltage-gated channels within the membrane that allow ions to flow across the membrane and transiently alter the membrane potential. A series of local circuits along the length of the cell then carry the action potentials along the neural membrane. If we were to transmit action potentials through the cytoplasm of the nerve (known as 'axoplasm'), instead of by local circuits along the membrane, messages could not be carried more than a few millimetres as axoplasm is actually quite a bad conductor of electricity.

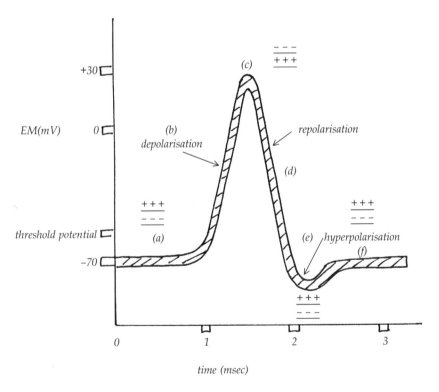

(a) Resting membrane potential.
(b) Opening of Na⁺ voltage-gated channels.
(c) Na⁺ channels start closing due to time dependency, K⁺ start opening.
(d) K⁺ channels opening, Na⁺ channels shutting.
(e) Na⁺ channels shut still same K⁺ open.
(f) Back to normal, K⁺ shut.

Fig. 5.3 An action potential.

Transmission of action potentials

Action potentials are generated in the initial segment of the axon known as the axon hillock. They are generated because the membrane potential (Em) of the cell body of the nerve (soma) has been depolarised by a stimulus reaching the fine input fibres or dendrites. There are two main types of axon, myelinated and unmyelinated.

Unmyelinated

The propagation of an action potential along an unmyelinated neurone occurs via local circuits (see Figure 5.4). Current flows in a circuit as shown in the diagram; by convention this is from positive to negative. Each local circuit acts as a stimulus for the next action potential. The very first part of the rising phase of the action potential is due to this local current. As the action potential spreads along the axon length, this changes the membrane potential at other points. Current also leaks out of the axon as it travels along the nerve; in other words, the initial depolarisation is attenuated with distance. However as long as the membrane potential remains greater than the threshold potential, another action potential will be stimulated.

Myelinated

This has a Schwann cell wrapped around the axon. Most nerve axons of vertebrates are myelinated. All motor axons are

(a)

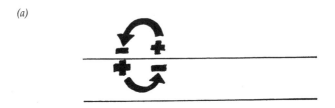

(b)   action
       potential

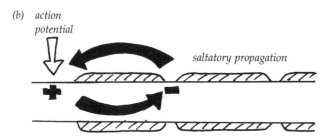

saltatory propagation

Fig. 5.4 Propagation of an action potential in: (a) an unmyelinated neurone, (b) a myelinated neurone.

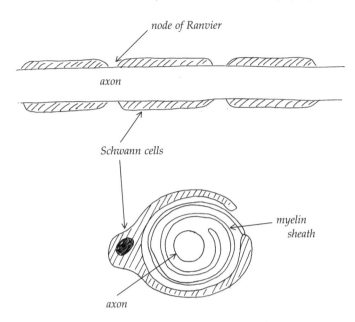

node of Ranvier

axon

Schwann cells

myelin sheath

axon

Fig. 5.5 Cross-section of a myelinated neurone.

myelinated. In myelinated nerves, the process is slightly more refined. The myelin sheath insulates the axon and stops leakage of current out of the axon. As there is less leakage, there is less attenuation and the action potential is carried further. Action potentials can only occur at nodes. This is called 'saltatory propagation' or jumping propagation as the signal jumps from one node to the next along the nerve, much more quickly than in an unmyelinated nerve.

Conduction velocities

In myelinated axons, conduction velocities are proportional to axon diameter. If the diameter of the axon is increased, the conduction velocity is increased. Conduction velocities in myelinated axons are around 120 m/sec or 432 km/h.

In unmyelinated axons, the conduction velocity is proportional to the square root of the diameter. There is not so much to be gained by increasing the diameter of the neurone in this case. Nerve impulses travel at around 0.5 m/s for unmyelinated nerves. Why not, then, have all nerves as myelinated nerves? Why should autonomic nerves and certain pain sensory fibres be unmyelinated? The simple, and rather dull answer, is that they would simply take up too much space and would not bring any real advantage.

Conduction velocities in all nerves are decreased by cold, around 3% of the maximum velocity is lost for each 1 degree Celsius drop in temperature. Cold impairs neural function and this is just as important to the horse as it is to us.

Effect of surrounding tissue

It should be clear by now that the transmission of nerve impulses efficiently and effectively is essential for the integration of behaviour. This transmission depends on nerves being activated as a result of relative changes in the charge differential across the membrane of these cells. The nature of the cellular environment surrounding the neurone is therefore critical. As we shall see a special barrier to ensure a constant environment protects the central nervous system. This does not extend to the peripheral nerves and so they may be more prone to the effects of general changes in the body such as those caused by over-exercise or certain metabolic diseases.

Receptor adaptation

Receptors vary in the duration of their response to a stimulus. Some receptors cause action potentials within the sensory nerve at the same rate the whole time the stimulus is present, in others, the

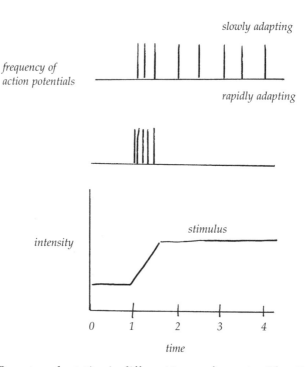

Fig. 5.6   Receptor adaptation in different types of receptor. The stimulus is as shown in the lower graph for both receptors, but results in a different pattern of release in the two types of receptor.

frequency of action potentials diminishes with time. The former are called 'slowly adapting receptors' and the latter, 'rapidly adapting receptors'. Receptors that respond to fine touch and pressure are rapidly adapting, whilst joint, muscle and pain receptors are slowly adapting. The rate of adaptation is thus suited to the function of the receptor. For example, if pain receptors were rapidly adapting, the animal would feel the pain but then the feeling would go away, so it would not be encouraged to take action to prevent further injury.

Receptor adaptation is one reason why an animal stops responding to a constant stimulus. Habituation, which is a learning process (see Chapter 9), will also result in a cessation of response to a constant stimulus. It is important to distinguish these processes, for example when you ask a horse to accept a saddle for the first time. If he habituates to the feeling, you will not have such a problem the next time you try to saddle the horse, but if the horse has merely accepted it because of sensory adaptation then the same behaviour can be expected the next time you try to saddle him.

The spinal cord

The spinal cord acts as a control centre, integrating incoming sensory information and producing appropriate motor output. It also acts as an intermediary nerve station between the peripheral nervous system and the brain, and forms the first level of information processing. The left and right halves of the spinal cord are symmetrical. In cross-section it is shaped like a butterfly, but the 'wings' are known as horns. The outside of the spinal cord is composed of white matter which is so called because it consists mainly of myelinated fibres in bundles, and the fat in the myelin makes it look white. The inner area is grey matter and is composed of nerve cell bodies, their processes, and numerous inter-neurones and their synapses. There are three functional zones along most of the spinal cord:

(1) Dorsal (posterior) horns   These contain sensory fibres i.e. this zone is concerned with input.
(2) Ventral (anterior) horns   These contain motor fibres.
(3) Middle   Here there is the association between sensory and motor fibres, i.e. it is concerned with information processing.

The white matter contains a number of nerve bundles, which link the spinal cord and the brain. If they contain sensory information going to the brain, they are called 'ascending fibres', if they contain motor information going to the spinal cord before reaching the periphery, they are called 'descending fibres'. The fibres come together in tracts.

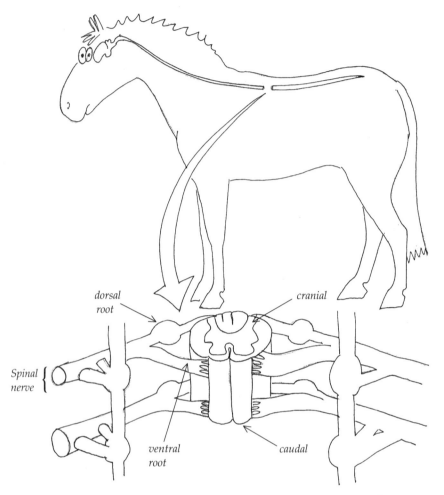

Fig. 5.7 Structure of the spinal cord of the horse.

Neuromuscular transmission

Motor nerves conduct impulses to the effector organs responsible for a response, where they form a synapse. As in the inter-neurone junctions, transmission of the impulse across the synaptic cleft is chemical, not electrical. Vesicles within the tips of the axon are full of transmitter substance. We will consider the case of a typical junction between a nerve and skeletal muscle in order to illustrate the general principles of the system. At such a neuromuscular junction the transmitter is acetylcholine (ach). Each vesicle contains about 10 000 molecules of acetylcholine which is synthesized locally in the terminal bouton of the nerve. At other types of junction, for example at those between nerves and smooth muscle, different transmitters, like noradrenaline, may be involved.

The synaptic cleft is about 50 nm wide and contains an enzyme called acetylcholinesterase. It takes acetylcholine about 0.5 msec to diffuse across the cleft to the motor end plate on the muscle fibre where it generates an end plate potential, which causes a succession of action potentials within the muscle fibre and ultimately a muscle contraction.

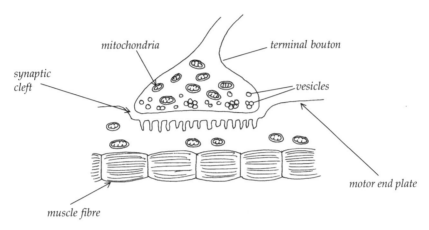

Fig. 5.8   A neuromuscular junction.

All muscles receive a certain amount of low level neural stimulation all the time. This is enough to give the muscle 'tone', so that it is ready for action when required. A certain amount of nerve input is necessary in order to keep the muscle healthy, and muscle without such a nerve supply will tend to wither away quite quickly. Even when a horse is just standing there is a constant stream of action potentials keeping the muscles at the right tension to hold the joints in the correct position against the forces of the horse's weight.

Nerve responses to transmitters

Synapses within the central nervous system can be either excitatory or inhibitory. The binding of neurotransmitter with receptor on the motor end plate in muscle always results in depolarisation of the membrane. The response of the motor end plate results in a move towards and beyond the threshold potential, i.e. there is an excitatory post-synaptic potential (EPSP). In other circumstances, stimulation of one nerve may actually inhibit a motor neurone. The change in membrane potential at the post-synaptic membrane is such that it moves away from the threshold potential, and so is less likely to fire an action potential. This is known as an inhibitory post-synaptic potential (IPSP). In other areas of the nervous system a combination of inhibitory and excitatory responses are used.

Usually many inter-neurones converge on one motor nerve and so the net effect of the sensory input on the motor neurone is the sum of all the inhibitory post-synaptic potentials and excitatory post-synaptic potentials that arrive at its post-synaptic membrane. This enables the body to produce grades of response and responses based on the overall picture rather than just simple knee-jerk style reflexes. Behaviour modifying drugs may affect the release, removal or binding of the transmitter as well as the generation of action potentials within a nerve. Their effects may therefore be quite widespread in the body.

Convergence of inter-neurones allows nerve nets or circuits to be built, which allow more complicated integration. In this situation a number of nerves all contribute to the probability of an action potential being generated in a focal cell. The advantage of this is that a low level of stimulation relating to several cells is capable of being recognised as similar to a higher level of stimulation of fewer cells. We will return to the importance of this when we discuss the functioning of the eye (see Chapter 6).

Central processing

Physical structure of the brain

The brain is an expanded part of the central nervous system involved in the integration of sensory information and the execution of appropriate motor responses. It is a fragile, jelly like structure, enclosed by membranous structures called meninges which line the bony brain-box (cranium) of the skull. In the spinal cord, most of the integration of information occurs deep within the tissue and so the grey matter is on the inside and the white matter on the outside. In the brain it is the other way round, so the white matter is on the inside and grey matter on the outside. There are, however, a few clusters of neurone cell bodies making up grey matter deep within the main body of the tissue. These grey matter regions are called nuclei (singular nucleus).

Brain tissue does not contain any blood vessels and so depends on the simple diffusion of nutrients from a sea of special fluid called cerebro-spinal fluid which surrounds it both inside and out. If the brain were a solid mass the central cells would never get enough oxygen and nutrients to survive. The cerebro-spinal canal, which carries the nutritious fluid within the core of the nervous tissue is expanded within the brain to form four ventricles, ensuring that active cells deep within the brain get a sufficient nutrient supply. One ventricle occurs in each cerebral hemisphere. These are called the lateral ventricles. The third ventricle is a tall slit in the mid-line between the two halves of the

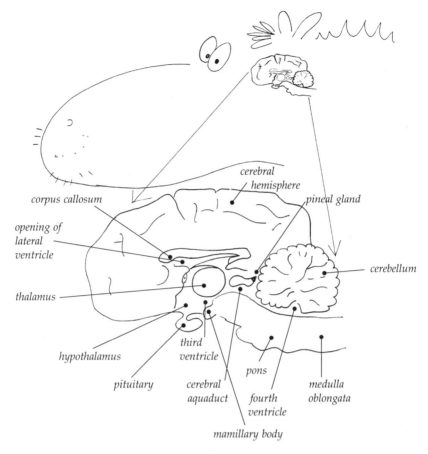

Fig. 5.9   Cross-section of the horse's brain.

thalamus and further back the fourth extends out sideways beneath the cerebellum.

There are a variety of classifications used to describe the brain. Typically, three regions are described:

(1)   **Forebrain** (telencephalon and diencephalon)
(2)   **Midbrain** (mesencephalon)
(3)   **Hindbrain** (metencephalon and myelencephalon).

The most obvious structures of the brain are:

(1)   **The cerebrum** (part of the forebrain)
(2)   **The cerebellum** (part of the hindbrain)
(3)   **The brain stem** (consisting of regions of fore-, mid-, and hindbrain).

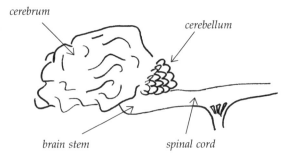

Fig. 5.10 Diagram of the external features of the brain.

The cerebrum or cerebral hemispheres

The cerebrum is the large egg-shaped structure at the front of the brain and consists of two important regions of grey matter in the horse, the cerebral cortex and the limbic system.

The cerebral cortex

The outermost folded layer is known as the cerebral cortex. It consists of only a thin layer of cells and is folded in order to increase its surface area. The ridges are called gyri (singular gyrus) and the grooves are called sulci (singular sulcus). It is involved in the integration of information relating to where the animal is in relation to the external environment. This includes visual, tactile, auditory and chemical information from the special senses, as well as general sensory information from the body surface and the position of the limbs etc. (proprioceptive information). It is also believed to be the place where the thinking for problem-solving occurs. There are specific lobes for these functions within the cortex:

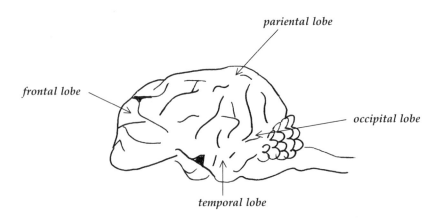

Fig. 5.11 Lobes of the cerebrum.

These lobes are associated with particular functions:

(1) **Frontal lobe** Planning and organisation of complex behaviours
(2) **Parietal lobe** Touch, pain, integration of the properties of an object and spatial orientation
(3) **Temporal lobe** Hearing, object recognition and recollection
(4) **Occipital lobe** Vision.

Limbic system

Deeper within the cerebrum is a collection of structures which form part of the limbic system, or emotional brain as it is sometimes known. Of these, the hippocampus and amygdala are involved in emotional behaviour, whilst the basal nuclei (caudate nucleus, putamen and globus pallidus) play an important role in regulating muscle tone and in initiating motor responses.

Linking the two halves of the cerebrum is a distinct area of white matter called the corpus callosum.

The cerebellum

Behind the cerebrum is a smaller structure which looks a bit like a cauliflower. This is the cerebellum. It is responsible for co-ordination of fine movements, the maintenance of balance and complex motor patterns.

The brain stem

The brain stem in the main trunk of tissue lying underneath the structure described above. There are four main parts to it.

The medulla

The part continuous with the spinal cord is called the medulla and is largely made up of ascending and descending tracts (see above) and the nuclei relating to the last seven of the twelve pairs of cranial nerves. These nerves relay information between the tissues of the head and viscera of the body to the brain. Specifically, the vagus nerve (cranial nerve X) relays information concerning the viscera of the thorax and abdomen; the vestibulo-cochlear nerve (VIII) brings sensory information from the ear, the facial nerve (VII) serves the facial area; whilst the glossopharyngeal (IX) and hypoglassal nerves (XII) serve the base of the tongue and throat. Also in this region of the brain is a complex web of nervous tissue called the reticular formation, which actually extends further forward into another part of the brain stem called the pons. This reticular formation is vital to the control of respiration and the cardiovascular system.

The pons
The pons contains part of the reticular formation and the nuclei of the cranial nerve V (the trigeminal nerve which serves the front of the tongue and jaw area).

The midbrain
Continuing on the under surface of the brain in front of the pons is the midbrain. This contains a number of important relay centres and the nuclei of two pairs of nerves responsible for the movement of the eye. There is also a small nipple like projection from the surface called the mammilary body. This is very important in the functioning of memory.

Thalamic region
The structure then continues into the thalamic and hypothalmic regions before disappearing into the cerebral regions. Extending down from the brain at this point is the pituitary gland (see Figure 5.10).

(1) **The pituitary** This used to be referred to as the 'Master Gland', when it was thought that the pituitary gland was the highest level of endocrine control. In fact it is itself controlled by the hypothalamus above it. Nevertheless, it plays a fundamental role in the regulation of many other endocrine glands.
(2) **The hypothalamus** This is the control centre for the maintenance of the internal environment. It effectively regulates the feelings of thirst and hunger. It is also the site of control for temperature regulation and diurnal rhythms, as well as being at the head of the endocrine and autonomic nervous systems.
(3) **The thalamus** Above the hypothalamus is the thalamus. It deals with the information coming from the cerebral cortex relating to the perception of the outside world. It interprets events in the external environment and initiates appropriate responses. Together the hypothalamus and the thalamus play an essential role in the motivation of behaviour.

Behavioural motivation

By understanding the function of the horse's brain, and appreciating in what respects it is similar and in what ways it is different to our own, we will get a better understanding of the horse's mind.

Horses have all the right structures to feel pain. We have all seen the physical manifestations of pain such as lameness, and have seen pain relief and improvement when painkillers are administered. There would seem to be no doubt that horses suffer from physical pain, and that the process is similar to that which occurs in humans.

But what about mental pain and suffering? The evidence here is much less clear. We may be fairly confident that we are doing good for our horse by providing for all of his physiological needs, with good food, warmth, fresh water, etc., but what are his mental needs? In order to understand this, it is not sufficient just to 'know about horses' and impose our preconceived ideas. We must try and learn what motivates them. Some aspects to this question will be discussed later in Chapter 10 on welfare.

Making decisions

In order to stay alive a horse must eat, drink, sleep, etc. These are his basic physiological needs. From evolutionary theory we can predict that horses which meet these needs more efficiently will be more successful and so leave more offspring. But what does efficiency mean in this circumstance? It means that a behaviour must effectively achieve its specific goal and that all the goals must be gathered with the minimum of cost. In other words, we can expect horses to have systems for working out what to do, how to do it and when it is best to do it. This involves balancing short-term needs with a long-term strategy. In order to do this efficiently, the brain must monitor current activity and the state of both the internal and external environments, it must then have some system for calculating its behavioural priorities. Motivation is concerned with the study of those factors which change the immediate priority status of an activity. In this context we use the term activity to describe the range of behaviours associated with achieving a particular goal or need. We could recognise two parts to such activities:

(1)   **Appetitive phase** An initial goal-seeking stage
(2)   **Consummatory phase** A final goal-achieving behaviour.

For example, a thirsty horse looking for somewhere to drink is performing appetitive behaviour. Once he has found the water and starts to drink he is performing consummatory behaviour. As he continues to drink, the motivation for this activity falls, a phenomenon known as 'negative feedback', and some other activity becomes his number one priority. The appetitive phase of the activity does not have such an effect on its motivation. If anything it increases it further; a phenomenon known as 'positive feedback'. In other words the longer an animal seeks the goal of a behaviour the harder it becomes for it to switch to doing anything else. Such a tendency stops animals from dithering or switching between behaviours so quickly that nothing gets done efficiently.

There are of course exceptions to these generalisations. Our thirsty horse may find a water source, but decide not to drink because there is a predator at the water hole. To do so at this time would endanger his life. In this case another short-term priority has intervened. Alternatively he may start to seek out water and, although not finding any, starts grazing instead. This is similar to the first example because as he looks for water and does not eat, so his need to feed increases as well. At some point it is possible that all this activity and lack of food means that feeding is now a bigger priority. The decision to switch to another behaviour involves two processes:

(1) Assessing all the factors contributing to the horse's need for water
(2) Considering the importance of the various other needs of the horse at that time.

A change in either or both of these may lead to a change in behaviour. So a horse may switch from one activity to another because:

(1) The goal for the first has been attained
(2) The importance of another behaviour increases because of an increase in the motivational factors affecting that behaviour.

There are two types of motivational factor:

(1) **Specific motivational factors** These only have a bearing on a specific behaviour. Specific motivational factors in our thirsty horse include the volume of body fluids and the concentration of body fluids.
(2) **General motivational factors** These affect the animal's tendency to perform a wide variety of behaviours. An example would be the level of arousal. If our horse is tired, it is not only unlikely to feel like drinking but also uninterested in playing, eating, or having sex. The state of arousal thus has an effect on a wide range of behaviour patterns.

Each activity then has its own set of motivational factors. Some are unique to that activity whilst others are shared with a broader range of behaviours. At any given moment a horse will have some motivation towards a number of behaviour patterns. We can represent this in what is known as a state space model as shown in Fig. 5.12.

On this plot two motivational states are considered, with the tendency to drink (thirst) on one axis and tendency to eat (hunger) on the other. The dominance boundary represents the point at which an animal will switch from one behaviour to another. When its level of hunger is plotted against its level of thirst and the mark falls above the line, point A, the horse will drink. If it falls below, e.g. points B or C, the horse will eat. The tendency to engage in a behaviour may be increased by either an increase in motivation for

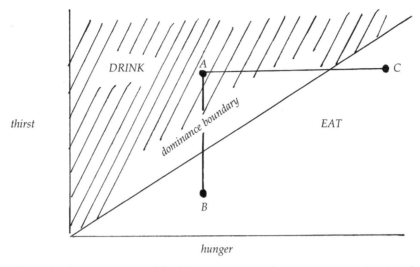

Fig. 5.12   State-space model of the competition between two motivational factors (motivation to eat and motivation to drink).

that behaviour (i.e. moving from A to C) or by a decrease in the motivation for competing behaviours (represented by movement from A to B). You will notice that in this instance, the horse does not need to get any hungrier for it to start eating, there is just a fall in thirst. This graph clearly shows that an animal's priorities are not fixed but depend on how well each demand is being met.

In domestication we decrease the motivation for foraging behaviour, as we provide our horses with readily accessible food. We should not be surprised then that other priorities become apparent which help to fill time. These may not be essential to living, but they may become the most important thing for the well-being of the animal's mental state. We will return to this theme later in the section on welfare (see Chapter 10).

So, in order to understand why an animal is doing something we must appreciate that this is an expression of the fact that the motivation factors for this behaviour are greater than those for any other. Therefore if we want a horse to do something else we may:

(1)   Reduce the motivation for the ongoing behaviour so that the next priority is expressed.
(2)   Specifically increase the motivation for the behaviour that we want.

Some behaviours like those associated with fears and phobias are largely governed by external causal factors and the motivation for these behaviours can be totally removed by eliminating the associated stimuli. Moreover the disappearance of these behaviours in captivity because of the absence of the causes is unlikely to cause a welfare problem in itself. Behaviours which are heavily dependent on internal causal factors, are more difficult to manage at the causal level. Internal psychological factors tend to be managed through training and psychotherapy (see Chapter 9) whilst internal physiological factors may be altered by medical or surgical intervention from a veterinary surgeon. These two categories of internal causal factor are not mutually exclusive as one affects the other. For example, drugs like antidepressants have a well defined physiological and psychological effect, and psychological stress has an enormous impact on the normal physiology of an individual as we shall see in Chapter 8. Our preference for a particular route to behaviour management should be based on consideration of the impact of the treatment on the well-being of the patient rather than sentiment for or against a particular therapy.

Autonomic and somatic nervous systems

We should not leave this section on the mechanisms of behaviour without some brief consideration of the mechanics of the output. The horse obviously has its own unique behaviour patterns as we shall see in Chapters 7 and 8, but the mechanics of these processes are broadly similar across most domestic species. There are two broad types of output from the central nervous system: autonomic and somatic.

The autonomic system

The autonomic nervous system is concerned with the control of the visceral organs of the body. It is that branch of the nervous system which controls heart rate, respiration rate, blood pressure, etc. Inputs of the autonomic nervous system come from both internal and external receptors; outputs of the autonomic nervous system are to smooth muscle which is found in the gut and blood vessels, cardiac muscle and glands. This autonomic output is itself divided into systems: the parasympathetic and sympathetic nervous systems.

Parasympathetic system

This part of the motor nervous system becomes active when the body is engaged in the processes relating to general body maintenance, such as eating and digesting food. It slows the heart and respiration rates, increases the blood supply to the gut and so forth. It calms things down within the body. The neuromuscular transmitter used in the synapses is acetylcholine.

Sympathetic system
This has the opposite effect to the parasympathetic nervous system. It speeds things up and gets the body ready for action. The heart beats faster when stimulated by the sympathetic nervous system, and the muscles in the blood vessels supplying the gut constrict so that less blood goes here and more to the skeletal muscles. The transmitter at the neuromuscular junction is noradrenaline, a very close relative of the hormone adrenaline which has similar properties. These hormones prepare the body for bursts of physical exercise, for example when about to take flight from a predator. This system becomes activated when an animal is stressed. It is designed to help the animal to deal with acute situations not chronic ones but is activated in both circumstances. This is one of the reasons why chronic stress can cause a lot of harm (see Chapter 10).

The somatic system

The somatic nervous system refers to the parts of those parts responsible for the movement of skeletal muscle. We have already discussed how the nerves here bring about action in the muscles of the body (see above). Some of these responses are initiated or co-ordinated at a spinal level, like the sequence of impulses required for locomotion, whereas others such as the co-ordination of the muscles for grooming originate in the brain. Some behaviour problems are controlled by intervention at this level. For example, cribbing may be 'treated' by cutting out the nerve that controls the muscles which facilitate this behaviour. This surgery has, at best, a variable success rate, does nothing to address the underlying causal factors and may in fact have a detrimental psychological impact. It should not therefore be considered as an easy option.

In summary, the autonomic and the somatic nervous systems share sensory nerves, but have very different motor systems, utilising different transmitters at the synapses and neuromuscular junctions.

TOPICS FOR DISCUSSION

◊ The disappearance of a behavioural response may be due to receptor adaptation, receptor fatigue or habituation. How could you distinguish between these?

◊ Why do behaviour modifying drugs so often have such broad side effects?

◊ As a result of exercise, the ionic composition of the tissue fluid surrounding peripheral nerves and muscles, may change. This can produce muscle cramps and twitches in the horse. What might happen if the barrier protecting the brain from these ionic changes was to fail?

◇ If horses need exercise what does this tell us about the motivation of the behaviour? What internal and external factors might have an effect on such a need?

◇ Compare and contrast the long- and short-term goals of a horse's existence.

◇ What is the difference between the physiological basis of behaviour and its psychological basis?

◇ Consider the nature of the changes which must occur centrally in order for there to be an alteration in the intensity of a response to a given stimulus (a quantitative change). Compare this to the changes required for a shift in the nature and type of response made to the same stimulus (a qualitative change).

References and further reading

Burt, A.M. (1993) *Textbook of Neuroanatomy*. W.B. Saunders, Philadelphia.

Goodenough, J., McGuire, B. & Wallace, R. (1993) *Perspectives on Animal Behaviour*. J.Wiley & Son, New York.

Guthrie, D.M. (1980) *Neuroethology: An Introduction*. Blackwell Scientific Publications, Oxford.

Guyton, A.C. (1991) *Basic Neuroscience: Anatomy and Physiology* 2nd edn. W.B. Saunders, Philadelphia.

von Holst, E. (1973) *The Behavioural Physiology of Animals and Man*. Methuen, London.

Kapit, W., Macey, R.I. & Meisami, E. (1987) *The Physiology Coloring Book*. Harper Collins, New York,.

Nathan, P. (1988) *The Nervous System*. Oxford University Press. Oxford.

Peters, R.S. (1958) *The Concept of Motivation*. Routledge & Kegan Paul, London.

Prosser, C.L. (1973) *Comparative Animal Physiology*, 3rd edn. W.B. Saunders, Philadelphia.

Swenson, M. & Reece, W. (1993) *Duke's Physiology of Domestic Animals* 11th edn. Cornell University Press, Ithaca.

Temple, C. (1993) *The Brain*. Penguin Books, London.

Toates, F. (1986) *Motivational Systems*. Cambridge University Press, Cambridge.

6. The Special Senses

The sensory homunculus is a picture of a human drawn from a proportional representation of the various areas of the body on the sensory cortex in the forebrain. The greater the sensory supply, the larger the organ on the homunculus, it therefore gives us an idea of the sensory priorities of the animal. The picture for a human is shown in Figure 6.1. We do not yet know what the picture would look like for horses, but we can hazard a guess at something approximating the horse in the same diagram. Amongst this supply there are a number of organs which are specifically involved in detecting certain features of the outside environment. These are the special sense organs of the eye, ear, nose and tongue.

Sight

Each eye consists of a layer of light receptors, (photoreceptors), a lens system that focuses light on these receptors, and a system of nerves that conducts impulses from the receptors to the brain. The eyes are rotated and moved synchronously by the action of seven muscles attached to the eyeball.

Horses' eyes are 5 × 6.5 cm in size and amongst the largest of any living mammal. This immediately suggests that the horse relies heavily on sight for information about the external environment.

Light rays pass through several media before they reach the photoreceptor cells. The first is the cornea which tends to bend the light rays inwards because of its curved surface. The rays then pass through the aqueous humour, between the cornea and the lens. On passing through the lens, the light rays are bent again, so that parallel rays entering the eye are bent inwards to a point called the focal point. Behind the lens is the vitreous humour, a transparent medium which helps the eyeball keep its shape.

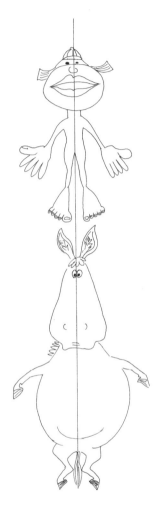

Fig. 6.1   Homunculus and the possible equine equivalent – an 'equunculus'!

Photoreceptors

There are two types of photoreceptor: namely rods and cones arranged on the sensitive layer of the eye known as the retina.

(1)   **Rods** are more responsive than cones to low light intensities, they only contain one pigment and so they can only send information relating to whether they are active or not. As a result the brain can only produce black and white images from their input. They allow night vision but not the recognition of colour in low light conditions.

(2)   **Cones** have several pigments which respond to different wavelengths of light, i.e. different colours. Each visible colour in the outside world produces a unique combination of activity amongst the pigments and so provides a code for the brain to recognise colour. These pigments are less sensitive than the

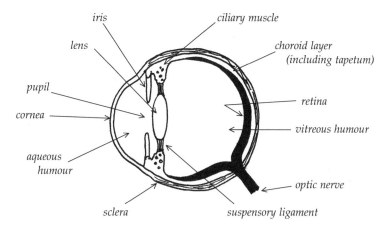

Fig. 6.2 Anatomy of the eye.

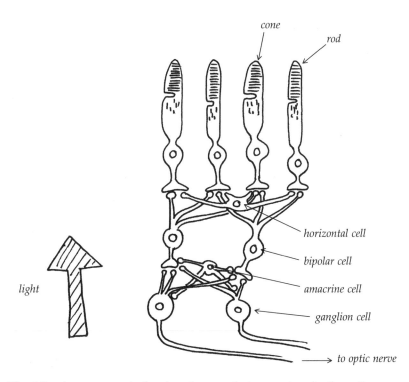

Fig. 6.3 Arrangement of rod and cone photoreceptors in the retina.

one found in rods and so colour vision is only possible when there is more light.

The visual world of the horse compared to our own

Field of view

Horses have a greater total field of view than humans but their perception of depth is less than ours.

In the horizontal plane horses can see nearly 360 degrees (see Figure 6.4). The exception is a blind spot behind the horse of about 5 degrees, which just about coincides with where a rider sits. Is it any wonder that horses are initially very wary about taking a rider on board? This area can be viewed by the horse when it raises or turns its head. Notice that raising the head and neck is a usual reaction to an alarming or interesting noise. It is pretty obvious that this wide field of view is an advantage to a prey animal, as he is more likely to be able to see predators approaching; it also means that he can keep an eye on the rest of the herd members more easily.

Each eye may have a field of view of up to 215 degrees in a plane parallel with the corners of the eye, but 190–95 degrees is more normal. There is obviously some degree of overlap in these fields so the brain receives two images (one from each eye) for some areas. This is known as the 'binocular field' and is the only area in which the horse has truly 3D (stereoscopic) vision and is able to judge distances accurately. It represents an arc of about 70 degrees at most in front of the horse and so we should not be surprised to find that horses are generally poor at judging distances. The 'monocular field' of view, that is the area covered by only one eye, is therefore about 290 degrees in total or 140–45 degrees on each side.

In the vertical plane each eye has a field of view of about 180 degrees.

The large visual field of the horse is due to the size and placement of the eyeballs. Placed laterally, they have a wide visual field, but this is at the expense of a smaller binocular field. The very round shape of the eyeball and its extensive lining with a sensitive retina also allow extreme peripheral vision. Those breeds which tend to have less protruding and more laterally placed eyeballs, e.g.

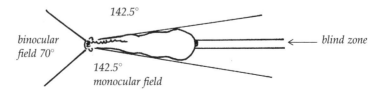

Fig. 6.4   Aerial view of a horse showing the extent of its field of vision.

Thoroughbreds and Standardbreds, have smaller visual fields and less stereoscopic capacity. Breeds with more forward pointing eyes or large bulbous eyes, like the Arab, probably have a more extensive binocular field within which they can accurately judge distances.

There are two main blind spots. One is directly behind the horse and consists of the area blocked by the width of the head and has an arc of about 5 degrees. The other is directly below his nose and is in more the vertical plane. As a result of this, a horse can not see a fence very well, if at all, as he is jumping it. He has to rely on the image of the fence that he receives one or two strides out. He can, however, get a better look at the fence with stereoscopic vision by tilting his head at the last moment and many horses can be seen to do this if they are unsure.

Objects appearing out of the blind spot directly behind a horse can startle them. People, who have no other knowledge of horses will have been taught 'Don't go round the back' as if to do so would almost certainly result in being kicked. In a stabled situation, it is not always possible to avoid this, but it is made safer by keeping a hand on the horse so that he has no reason to be startled by your sudden reappearance.

Vision in low light
Horses can see in lower light intensities than humans

The horse has a fibro-elastic layer beneath the retina lining the inside of the eye-ball. This structure is called a 'tapetum lucidum' and reflects light back onto the retina. A horse therefore makes better use of the available light and is better able to see in dim situations than a human. However this also means that horses are more easily blinded by brighter light and in part explains why they often have difficulty crossing between light and dark contrasting areas. This does not mean that the horse is nocturnal, but feral horses tend to be more active around dawn and dusk. Other structures which help the horse to function in low light levels include the sensitivity of the pigment in photosensitive cells and the relatively large size of the eye.

Most light entering the eye will come from the sky above, but the horse does not need to know much about what is going on above him as he does not naturally have aerial enemies. The efficiency of the eye is therefore improved by some of this light being shaded out. There are a number of ways in which the horse achieves this.

(1) The eyelashes act as a sun screen.
(2) Within the eye attached to the top margin of the pupil are some large cyst like structures. These are called the corpora nigra or iris bodies, it is believed that they too act like a set of internal light-screens within the eye.

(3)   The shape of the pupil also helps in this capacity, as it is broader than it is high. This decreases the light entering the eye from above and below but maintains the visual field in the horizontal plane.

Visual acuity

The visual acuity of the horse is less than that of a human and best along a wide axis.

Visual acuity is the degree to which the details and contrasts of colours are perceived. The amount of detail which can be determined is influenced by a range of factors, one of these being the density of photoreceptors. A greater density means that more detail can be picked out. Imagine the difference in clarity between a mosaic made out of tiny 1 mm pieces and the same picture made out of 1 cm blocks. Lying along the horizontal axis of the eye, there is a narrow region of the retina which has a particularly high photoreceptor density, with as many as 5000 cells per square millimetre. This is called the 'visual streak'. In people, it is a round focal spot but in the horse it is more of a wide band. Directly above and below this region, the density of photoreceptors (and hence the acuity), is less, so that objects viewed in these areas are not seen so clearly.

Other factors which affect the acuity of vision include the degree of convergence of photoreceptors onto the optic nerve. Several photoreceptors may converge on a single nerve cell in order increase its activity in low light, but input from a wider receptor field (see Chapter 5) reduces the acuity – in effect increasing the relative size of our pieces of mosaic.

High definition images also depend on sharp focus. This a function of the flexibility of the lens and the strength of the muscles which change its shape (ciliary muscles). As the muscles contract they flatten the lens and so bend the incoming light less. This means the horse can focus on more distant objects (see Figure 6.5). It seems that the horse's lens system is not very flexible and tends to be fixed on long distance focus. This means that it is not easy for the horse to focus on objects which are very close. However, it does seem that horses are quite capable of discriminating quite complex patterns and different faces.

Horses tend to throw their heads up to see objects at close range particularly when startled. This is probably done in order to try to focus the object onto the visual streak in order to get a good clear view of it.

Long-sight

Horses are 'long-sighted' compared to humans.

Walls (1942) suggested that horses had a 'ramped' retina and

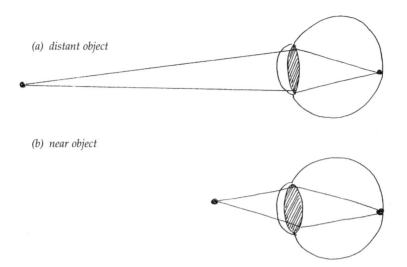

(a) *distant object*

(b) *near object*

Fig. 6.5 A different shaped lens is required for focussing near versus distant objects. For near objects the lens is more rounded so that the light rays can be bent more.

used a static mechanism for focusing objects at different distances, a process known as accommodation. This meant that they would tend to focus near objects at the top and bottom of the retina and distant object along the main optical axis where the distance was shorter. In order to bring near objects into view, the horse would have to move his head up or down. Prince *et al.* (1960) suggested that this was in addition to the more conventional dynamic ciliary muscle accommodation system. In 1975, Sivak and Allen demonstrated that the retina was not ramped after all, and that the horse was only capable of dynamic accommodation. It appears that the horse's eye 'at rest' as it were, is naturally focussed on more distant objects than our own eyes. In other words, horses are long-sighted compared to humans. This is probably an adaptive trait, since the horse in open grassland is most concerned with discerning whether or not distant objects are in fact predators. By the time they get close, it is probably getting a bit late!

Colour vision
Horses cannot distinguish between colours as well as humans can.

In order to have full colour vision an animal needs three types of visual pigment. This is located in the photoreceptor cones. Each responds optimally to a different wavelength of light (colour) but reacts to some degree to a much broader range of wavelengths. There should be considerable overlap between the sensitive range of the pigments. Humans have three different types of pigment,

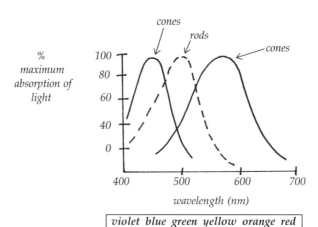

Fig. 6.6   Absorption spectra of rods and cones.

responding maximally to light at wavelengths of 440, 540, and 565 nm, corresponding to blue, green and red respectively. One type of cone on its own would be no good, as it is recognising the difference in response of each type of cone that produces a colour perception. If there are only two pigments some colour blindness is possible. This is a difficult area of study and if controls are inadequate, false conclusions may be reached.

Grzimek (1952) performed a colour perception test, by training horses to go to different coloured buckets for food reward. The results suggested that horses could discriminate between colours and between 27 shades of grey. Prior to this, it was thought that horses were completely colour blind. The horses in this experiment distinguished yellow most easily, followed by green, blue and finally red, suggesting that they possessed three pigments similar to humans.

Pick *et al.* (1994) repeated Grzimek's work, using additional controls for auditory, olfactory, tactile and positional cues which might have affected Grzimek's results. Their results suggested that horses could discriminate between shades of blue and red, but could not discriminate green from a grey of the same brightness. Their conclusion was that horses had some colour vision, but only two pigments, i.e. that their vision was dichromatic; horses were colour blind to green because it stimulates both red and blue cones weakly, and therefore it cannot be distinguished from whites or greys. Also at either end of the spectrum, where only one cone is stimulated by the light, it is probably harder for the horse to differentiate between shades. However the issue of colour blindness in the horse remains unresolved (see Macuda & Timney 1999, and Smith & Goldman 1999).

Peripheral vision

Horses are very sensitive to objects moving on the periphery of their field of vision.

It is likely that movement along the edge of the field of vision may be accentuated in horses. This is particularly due to a heightened sensitivity of ganglion nerve cells towards the periphery of the retina. In the wild, horses respond to predators if they come too close or if they suddenly move and so sensitivity to movement is an important survival trait. The detection of movement also helps identify a camouflaged potential predator.

Sudden or stilted movements therefore alert horses and may cause anxiety. This can cause problems if even a familiar person suddenly appears or moves in the horse's field of view. We can, however, use this trait to our advantage. Sudden and rigid movements can be used when free-schooling in order to get the horse to focus its attention in our direction. This is one of the principles to the popular 'join up' technique discussed in Chapter 9.

The visual world of the horse is very different to our own and we should avoid imposing our own perceptions on an explanation of what he sees happening. By understanding his special sensitivities and weaknesses we can work with him and train him more effectively.

Hearing

The equine ear is a complex three chambered structure involved not only with receiving auditory signals but also sending visual ones. The mobility of the ears is important in localising sound and may indicate in which direction a horse's attention is focused. Lowering of the ears is used as a threat but may also be part of a submissive gesture. We will start our consideration of this multifunctional structure with an account of its anatomy.

Anatomy of the ear

The external ear

This consists of the earflap (pinna) and a connecting cartilage (annular cartilage). The funnel shape helps focus sound waves onto the ear drum within. The movement of each pinna is controlled by sixteen muscles, which can operate independently. The horse is therefore capable of a dual focus in attention. When the ears are laid back the ear canal may be almost completely closed so the horse can hear little at this time.

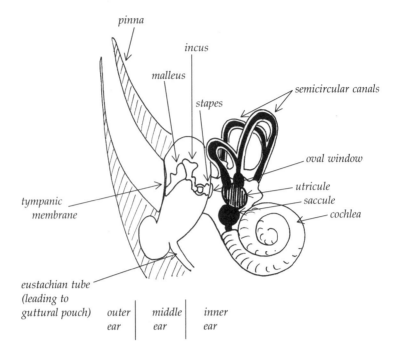

Fig. 6.7 Anatomy of the ear.

The middle ear

This consists of a chamber separated from the external ear by the ear drum or tympanic membrane. It contains three bones (the malleus, incus and stapes, otherwise known as the hammer, anvil and stirrup), which transfer and amplify the vibration of the tympanic membrane onto the inner ear.

A short tube, the eustachian tube, connects the middle ear to the back of the pharynx. This ensures that the pressure in the middle ear is the same as that outside. If this is not the case, sound waves are not accurately conducted to the sensitive regions of the inner ear. The guttural pouch is an expanded region of this tube around the back of the jaw. Its function still remains a mystery.

The inner ear

This contains the cochlea, with its auditory sensitive cells and the vestibular apparatus (the utricle, semicircular canals and saccule), which are important in balance. The auditory sensitive cells convert sound waves into electrical messages for transmission to the brain.

Hearing

Sound waves are produced by particles vibrating in a physical medium, e.g. air, water or a solid. Sound cannot travel in a vacuum.

Sound waves are perceived in terms of their loudness and their pitch, corresponding to the amplitude and frequency of the wave. Not all sound wave detection is interpreted as noise, and not all sound waves are detected by the ear. The vibrissae (whiskers) around the muzzle and even the hooves are thought to detect vibrational energy to a certain extent, since these structures have suitable rapidly adapting mechanoreceptors.

Amplitude or loudness

Loudness is the intensity of a sound. It is measured in decibels (dB), with 3 dB corresponding to a whisper and 130 dB corresponding to a jet engine.

Horses are better than man at discriminating between noises of similar loudness. They appear to be able to discriminate between a single decibel for certain sounds within the range 69–70 dB (Popov cited by Rees, 1984).

Horses can protect their ears from very loud noise by laying their ears flat in order to close down the auditory canal. So a horse that lays its ears back in response to a loud noise may not be scared, simply trying to protect itself. Similarly a horse may lay its ears back if you shout at it. In this circumstance it is important to look at the whole picture in order to see whether or not the horse is simply trying to protect its hearing, is scared or is being aggressive.

Frequency or pitch

High frequency sound waves produce high pitched noises and low frequency produces low pitched noises. Frequency is measured in Hertz (Hz). Our range of hearing (when it is at peak performance as children) extends from around 20 Hz to 20 kHz, but the horse can hear from 60 Hz to around 33.5 kHz (Heffner & Heffner 1985). It is therefore capable of hearing many high pitched sounds (ultrasound) to which we are oblivious but does not hear with its ears the lower frequencies that we do. Sensitivity to ultrasound is believed to help in the localisation of a noise. Since the soft tissue of the head readily blocks such noise, the ear nearest to the source will receive more high frequency sounds. The horse has its greatest sensitivity to sound at around 2 kHz, but it requires louder sounds than a human at even this frequency. Some sounds which we can hear, therefore, the horse will not detect. The optimal range of between 2–5 kHz includes the range of frequent equine calls and, fortunately for us, most human speech as well.

Anecdotal reports suggest that horses can detect very low frequencies, e.g. the geophysical vibrations preceding earthquakes, and it has been suggested that these are not 'heard' as such but may be detected by the hoof.

Localisation of sound

Most animals find it easier to localise sound in the horizontal plane than the vertical plane. To determine where a sound is coming from, the signal received by each ear is compared. If a sound comes from a source to the right of the horse, it will be louder in that ear than the left, it will reach it sooner and it will contain more high frequency noise. In other words, there will be:

(1)   an inter-aural amplitude difference
(2)   an inter-aural time difference
(3)   an inter-aural spectral difference.

By comparing the signals from the two ears, the brain is able to work out where the sound is coming from. Fraser (1992) suggests that in addition to these mechanisms, a horse facing the source of a sound, receives a reflected signal from the shoulders. There is then in effect a rapid echo with an inter-aural delay. If such a system were employed it would allow the accurate location of sound in three dimensional space. To date the available experimental evidence does not support such a hypothesis. Whilst humans are able to locate a sound within about a degree the horse has a threshold of around 25 degrees. This is a little better than the cow but a lot worse than most carnivores who depend heavily on sound localisation for their hunting.

In response to a novel sound, horses can be seen to engage in a graded response depending on the level of interest. First one ear turns towards the source, then the other as well, beyond this the head is turned and ultimately the horse may orientate its whole body towards the sound.

Chemoreception

There are three main organs with external chemical receptors. These consist of:

(1)   The nerve endings in the main olfactory epithelium of the nose
(2)   Nerve receptors in the vomeronasal organ within the hard palate
(3)   Gustatory receptors (taste buds) on the tongue.

The functions of these receptors are:

(1)   To identify and signal the presence of specific chemicals
(2)   To signal the concentration of specific chemicals.

On the basis of this information certain behaviours and physiological changes are initiated. Because humans have such a poor sense of smell and virtually no vomeronasal organ we tend to underestimate the importance of this sense.

Smell

The olfactory system
The sense of smell depends upon the ability to detect and interpret airborne chemicals (olfaction). This information is relayed from the nasal region to the brain by the paired olfactory nerves known as the first cranial nerves (I). Horses have an extensively folded sensory area over the back of the nasal cavity (the cribriform plate) and so have a much more extensive sense of smell than we do. The sensation of flavour is closely linked to the integration of olfactory and gustatory stimulation. Even with our limited sense of smell we have experienced how food seems tasteless when we have a heavy cold.

The receptor structure of the nose
The horse's long nose provides a large surface area for the olfactory mucosa and this is made larger by the folding of structures such as the cribriform plate. The receptor cells are modified bipolar neurones with tiny hair-like projections called cilia extending beyond the surface of the mucosa. These structures contain receptors which bind with individual molecules and multiply the sensitivity of the surface even more. Input from these cells is ultimately relayed to the cortex of the brain where conscious perception occurs and to the limbic system, which is associated with more emotional behaviour. The receptors are relatively rapidly adapting nerve cells and so it would seem that it is the detection of new chemicals in the environment which is most important rather than the continuous monitoring of air quality. Whilst sniffing increases the intake of chemical laden air, the process of snorting is thought to help clear the sensory areas so that the next inhalation presents a true impression of the current aerial environment.

The vomeronasal organ
This was first described by Jacobson in the early 19th century, and is sometimes referred to as Jacobson's organ. It is found in many mammals, but in man is reduced to a shallow pit inside the nose. In the horse the vomeronasal organ consists of two blind ending tubes, approximately 12 cm long, lying either side of the nasal septum within the hard palate and towards the anterior part of the nasal cavity. They are highly vascular, cartilaginous structures with a mucous membrane lining. Communication with the nasal cavity is via the naso-palatine duct. The structure is innervated by sensory fibres of the main olfactory nerves, which travel directly without a synapse to regions of the limbic system. It therefore provides a direct route between certain chemicals in the environment and specific behavioural reactions. It seems that the presence of

potentially exciting chemicals is first detected by the main olfactory epithelium. This then encourages the horse to engage in a behaviour known as flehmen, or 'lip curl', which concentrates chemicals into the vomeronasal organ.

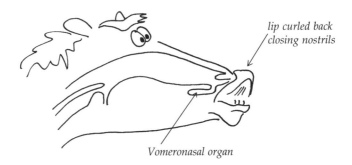

lip curled back
closing nostrils

Vomeronasal organ

Fig. 6.8   The vomeronasal organ and flehmen response.

All mammals with a vomeronasal organ show some sort of flehmen response. The characteristic action is associated with the detection of smells. When interesting, odour-filled air enters the nasal cavity as the horse inhales, the nasal chambers are closed by curling the lip back, 'trapping' the odour within the nares or nostril area. Movement of the tongue against the soft palate and champing of the jaw whilst in this position encourages the movement of air into the vomeronasal organ for sampling. The chemical also becomes dissolved in the nasal secretions, partly produced by the vomeronasal organ, and these probably flow along the organ as the head is tipped back. Flehmen is most common in mature stallions, but is seen in adult and juvenile horses of all sexes.

The vomeronasal organ is certainly important in the control and co-ordination of sexual activity, but it is probably involved in controlling a wider range of emotional behaviours, possibly including some forms of anxiety. If horses can smell chemicals associated with fear or alarm, it is likely that this is the organ responsible for their detection.

The vomeronasal organ may also be responsible for triggering certain maturational changes in the horse. In other species, the absence of female urine during the rearing of all-male groups can result in a reduced body weight and poor development of secondary sexual characteristics. Similarly, the absence of males during the development of females has been shown to delay puberty. Both of these effects are thought to be mediated by the vomeronasal organ.

Taste

Taste (gustation) is important to animals and affects their behaviour in a number of ways:

(1)   It allows an animal to discriminate between various foods. If a food with a novel flavour is associated with an animal feeling ill, any food with a similar taste is avoided in future. Unlike other forms of learning this association need only occur once for it to have a lasting effect. Certain plants like buttercups are obviously unpleasant to taste and avoided by horses.

(2)   It may provide information about the nutritional value of a food. Salt is a precious nutrient in the diet which is often in short supply. It seems that some taste receptors are specifically adapted to detecting this chemical so a horse may be able to ensure that it has sufficient salt in its diet by monitoring its intake through taste. Other 'nutritional wisdoms' may also exist, allowing an animal to choose a balanced diet when a range of foodstuffs is available.

(3)   Taste regulates digestion by influencing other aspects of gastro-intestinal physiology, for example by stimulating gastro-intestinal enzymatic secretions.

(4)   Taste also influences intake. Intake is greater in a horse for the more preferred foodstuffs such as timothy grass, dandelion and white clover. This suggests that feeding behaviour is not just concerned with the maintenance of the body's chemical balance (homeostasis) but incorporates hedonic aspects as well.

The regulation of intake also depends to a varying degree on learned factors associated with familiarity; horses may refuse to drink water which is not from their normal source or which is in a different container. This can cause problems in the horse which needs to be hospitalised. Home water, including buckets, should be provided. Alternatively the water may be sweetened to improve intake.

Gustatory receptors

Taste receptors are grouped into structures known as taste buds. These have tiny pores, from which microvilli project. Action potentials are formed within the taste cells when chemicals bind to these microvilli. Taste buds are mainly found on the tongue, but have been found on the anterior region of the soft palate, and the oral surface of the epiglottis. Buds are themselves organised into larger visible structures called papillae.

Papillae take on various morphological forms, with different types characteristic of certain regions of the tongue:

(1)   **Fungiform** (mushroom-like) papillae on the front of the tongue

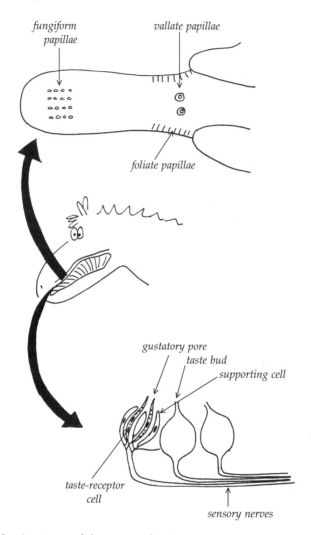

Fig. 6.9   Anatomy of the sense of taste.

(2)   **Vallate** (valley-like) papillae at the back of the tongue
(3)   **Foliate** (flower-like) papillae on the sides of the tongue.

Glands found between and at the bottom of the papillae secrete fluids that rinse the region, including the microvilli of the buds.

The lingual branch of the trigeminal (V) and glossopharyngeal (IX) cranial nerves innervate taste buds on the tongue according to their location.

In man there are four basic types of taste. These are sour, bitter, salt and sweet. It is likely that horses detect similar qualities (or 'sensory modalities' as they are also known) although there are almost certainly some differences since horses will drink solutions of sucra-octa acetate which we would find far too bitter. However, Randall *et al.* (1978) using taste preference tests in foals found the following with regard to each sensory modality:

(1) **Sour** Acetic acid solutions were rejected at concentrations above 0.16 ml/100 ml, and pH 2.9.
(2) **Salt** Foals were indifferent to salt at concentrations < 0.63 g/ 100 ml, or 0.63%, and rejected salt solutions above that concentration.
(3) **Sweet** Sucrose solutions were preferred to tap water at concentrations ranging from 1.25 to 10 g/100 ml, but foals were indifferent to concentrations above and below this.
(4) **Bitter** Quinine was rejected by foals at concentrations above 20 mg/100 ml.

Sensitivity to various taste types varies over the tongue; for instance, in man, the tip of the tongue is most sensitive to sweet tastes. This does not correspond with the type of papillae found in the various regions. No such information is available for the horse. Taste sensitivity and preference also varies greatly between individuals, as various factors (including nutritional status, electrolyte status, individual preference, previous experience and novelty) all contribute to the taste selections that horses make. Our own research over the last few years (Murphy *et al.* unpublished data) has demonstrated that horses may be trained to accept solutions which they would normally reject, by starting at low concentrations and gradually increasing the concentration of the otherwise unpalatable chemical. In this way it may be possible to ensure that horses are in an optimal electrolytic state before they compete. It is to be hoped that this will help to lead to the prevention of problems associated with ion imbalance following hard work and facilitate the more rapid restoration of ion balances during endurance work.

Cutaneous sensation

Whilst the skin is not a discrete organ for detecting a specific feature of the environment, it is nonetheless an important sensory structure. It therefore warrants a short description in this section. Sensitivity varies all over the body according to things like the thickness of the coat, the thickness of the skin, and the number of receptors at different points in the skin. Specific receptors in the skin detect heat, cold, touch, pressure, vibration and pain. The receptors for heat and cold are known as thermoreceptors, those for touch, pressure and vibration are mechanoreceptors, and those for pain or noxious stimuli are nociceptors. The level of tactile sensitivity may be gauged by the degree of innervation of the hair follicles of an area.

By this measure, it appears that the whiskers, and the long stiff hairs surrounding the eyes are particularly sensitive. The neck, withers, shoulders, coronets, rear of pastern and lower flank are also well innervated.

Cutaneous stimulation not only relays information relating to the particular sensory modality stimulated but may also change the level of arousal of the individual. Gentle stroking, particularly of the withers and crest seems to cause a slowing in the heart rate and the release of naturally soothing chemicals. This may explain why close associates in the field groom each other (see Chapter 7). Skin receptors have a relatively low threshold of stimulation for the modality for which they are best adapted, but will respond to other modalities at higher levels of stimulation. Over stimulation of any receptor type may be represented centrally as pain. The importance of touch in the horse for communication and control should not be underestimated but, scientifically, this is a relatively unexplored area.

TOPICS FOR DISCUSSION

◇ Consider the ecology of the senses in the horse.
◇ Is there an alternative explanation for the supposed extra-sensory perception (ESP) of some horses?
◇ What is the difference between sensation and perception?
◇ Compare the sensory biases of man with those that may occur in the horse. How might some of these lead to apparent management problems?
◇ Discuss the behaviours associated with the use of the various special sense organs of the horse.
◇ How would you design an experiment to assess whether or not horses are colour-blind? What controls would you need?

References and further reading

Fraser, A.F. (1992) *The Behaviour of the Horse*. CAB International, Wallingford.

Grzimek, B. (1952) Versuche uber das farbsechen von pflanzenessern. I. Das farbige sehen (und die Sehscharfe) von Pferden. *Zeitschrift fur Tierpsychologie* **9**, 23–39.

Heffner, R.S. & Heffner, H.E. (1983) Hearing in large mammal; horses (*Equus caballus*) and cattle (*Bos taurus*). *Behavioural Neuroscience* **97**, 299–309.

Heffner, R.S. & Heffner, H.E. (1985) Hearing in mammals: The least weasel. *Journal of Mammology* **66**: 745–55.

Macuda, T. & Timney, B. (1999) Luminance and chromatic discrimination in the horse (*Equus caballus*). *Behavioural Processes* **44**, 301–307.

Pick, D.F., Lovell, G., Brown, S. & Dail, D. (1994) Equine color perception revisited. *Applied Animal Behaviour Science* **42**, 61–5.

Prince, J.H., Diesem, C.D., Eglitis, I. & Ruskell, G.L. (1960) *Anatomy and Histology of the Eye and Orbit in Domestic Animals*. Thomas, Springfield.

Randall, R.P., Schurg, W.A. & Church, D.C. (1978) Responses of horses to sweet, salty, sour and bitter solutions. *Journal of Animal Science* **47**, 51–5.

Rees, L. (1984) *The Horse's Mind*. Stanley Paul, London.

Sivak, J.G. & Allen, D.B. (1975) An evaluation of the 'ramp' retina of the horse eye. *Vision Resarch* **18**, 1353–7.

Smith, S. & Goldman, L. (1999) Color discrimination in horses. *Applied Animal Behaviour Science* **62**, 13–25.

Walls, G.L. (1942) *The Vertebrate Eye and its Adaptive Radiation*. Cranbrook Institute of Science, Bloomfield Hills.

7. Communication and Social Organisation

Most horses tend to live in social groups when given the opportunity. This reflects their social nature. However, living successfully and peacefully with such a group depends on using the right signals (outputs) as well as understanding this language. We cannot realistically expect horses to learn our language and so we must try to understand theirs if we are to get the most out of our relationship with them. This involves understanding both the specific signals used and the nature of social organisation.

Communication

The development of the equine language

Communication is the transfer of a signal from one individual to another with the consequence that it affects the behaviour of the receiver. The two parties are mutually adapted for the process. It therefore has three important components.

(1) The signal sent by the sender
(2) The means of transfer (channel) used for the information exchange
(3) The message received by the receiver.

Communication not only identifies an individual, its activity and status but also is essential for the co-ordination of group activity.

When studying communication and communication problems it is important to examine and make sense of each of the components described above. Any explanation must answer questions like the following: how could the signal have evolved in the sender and how could its interpretation have evolved in the receiver?

For example, take the sexual display of the horse (see Chapter 8). In this display, the stallion gathers himself up, arches his neck and prances in front of a mare with a characteristic high stepping gait, like a piaffe. The mare stands, urinates small amounts of urine with chemical signals about her sexual state and rhythmically pushes out

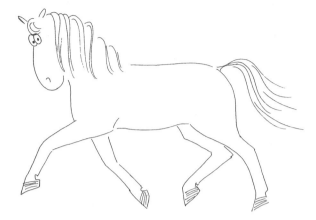

Fig. 7.1   Displaying stallion.

her clitoris (winking (see Figure 8.2)). Why should they go through this ritual? The stallion's display could be an incidental feature of how he feels in these circumstances. He is very excited but somewhat fearful because if the mare is not fully receptive she might cause quite a severe injury. The arching of the neck and tucking in of the head may help to focus on the mare close by (see Chapter 6). The mare's behaviour probably also reflects her current state of arousal.

When an animal gets very excited the sympathetic nervous system is activated and the bladder is emptied – no point in carrying extra weight if you are going to have to run for your life. Now imagine a mutation arose which meant that a specific chemical was released when a mare was ready to conceive. Those stallions that could smell the chemical and tried to mate at this time would be more successful and leave more offspring. The ability to produce and detect the chemical would therefore be heavily selected for. Within a comparatively small number of generations those animals which did not carry this trait would not breed so successfully and leave fewer offspring. In fact one might soon start to see selection favouring not just the ability to produce this chemical but the ability to produce and detect it ever more efficiently. Mares who produced it in their urine and who urinated when approached by a stallion sent a stronger and more efficient signal than those who did not display this behaviour. Pushing out the clitoris may be associated with voiding the last drops of urine but may incidentally help make the signal even clearer. So much so that those stallions who were attracted to this visual display from afar, even in the absence of the chemical (perhaps because of the distance or wind direction) would again be more successful breeders than those who could only respond to the chemical signal at close quarters. Anatomical and physiological changes which emphasise this behaviour in the mare when she is in oestrus, or its recognition in the stallion, then become an advantage in the competition to breed efficiently and success-fully. Clitoral winking then becomes an important sign in itself quite apart from the fact that it served a useful physiological function. The original function may now be redundant to the pro-cess but was vital to the evolution of the ritual language. Natural selection and evolution, which alters the attractiveness of one sex to the other in this way, is known as sexual selection (see Chapter 2).

Both parties should be willing for the most successful unions and the importance of female choice and preference should not be underestimated in shaping the form and behaviour of stallions. Another example of sexual selection may explain why most stal-lions have such a well-developed crest. If arching of the neck, as part of a stallion's display is attractive to mares at the time of mating, anything that emphasises this may improve a stallion's success. The preference of females for mates with more rounded necks then leads to selection favouring crested males.

But why should such signals and ritual displays be of any importance or attractive to a mare? Choice of a mate based on a limited number of features related to the anatomy and behaviour of a partner in courtship is as reliable and efficient a technique as any for assessing their genetic fitness. If the development of a crest is dependent on male hormone levels in the male, then choosing to mate with stallions with clear and unambiguous crests may help ensure that it is not a waste of time. The degree of perfection in the piaffe of the prancing stallion may reflect his bodily fitness and anatomical perfection. It is an important benchmark against which all stallions can be compared and judged. The effective force behind this demand is that a sick or injured horse cannot display so fluently. Natural selection favours the perfection of movement in these displays which is why they are such a joy to watch.

This type of explanation is favoured for the origin of commu-nicative signals in the horse because it fits within the theory of evolution and shows a clear fitness advantage to both sender and receiver in the development of such signals. The message can be detected and understood by the receiver at all stages of develop-ment and the channels used are optimal for the type of message sent. Specific features develop as a result of selection for more efficient ways of sending and receiving the information.

Understanding the language of another species

Most communication has evolved to occur between members of the same species (intra-specific communication) but this does not mean that understanding it is limited to this population. Many animals recognise the alarm calls of other species, especially if they share a common predator. There is an obvious biological advantage to this trait; an individual that is capable of acting on such a signal will have a head start when it comes to escape. This recognition of signs of alarm and fear probably extends to the horse and human. People who are nervous around horses signal their fear in many ways including their body language, and possibly smell – undetectable by humans. The horse may recognise this fear but not identify the cause of the problem, i.e. itself. It becomes nervous and this scares the novice even more. Eventually, unable to find any other cause of the problem, the horse may react by either trying to remove the source of its fear, the nervous horseman, or else the horse may panic. This is most likely if the horse is confined, as it has no way of using its preferred solution, which is to run away from the problem. At best the fears of each are confirmed and at worst serious injury to either or both may result.

The basis of effective training is effective communication and we must make sure that we also can make ourselves clear when we wish to communicate something to our horse. Since we are the ones with the more flexible problem-solving brains, it is our responsibility to analyse the situation and sort out the problem when things go wrong. It should not be the horse's job to learn to read our minds.

Just because most communication is directed to members of the same species, we should not assume that every member of the species would necessarily understand intra-specific signals. Animals that have been historically and evolutionarily isolated may have evolved their own variants on a theme. Little work has been done on this subject but it may represent the basis of a number of social problems like aggression within a group of horses which are strangers to each other, although there are often many other explanations which need considering in relation to this problem.

Effective communication depends on the signal being understood by the receiver, and we must always be prepared to examine this issue when things go wrong. If one horse does not understand the signal of another, confusion and aggression may result. Domestication can bring great variety to a species as a result of genetic changes and rearing conditions. It may be that different breeds place more emphatic importance on particular parts of the wild repertoire, or that rearing a young animal in isolation of a range of adults deprives it of the opportunity to learn the full repertoire. In either situation there is the potential for a new group member to fail to react appropriately to the signals of the group. This may then result in more overt gestures including aggression.

Do horses ever lie to us?

In order to lie an animal must be capable of deception. This does not mean that it needs to be evil. A range of species has shown the ability to manipulate the behaviour of others through the use of false signals.

(1)   Some types of manipulation are based on simple rules, which could have a genetic basis – evolutionary deception, e.g. the yellow and black hover fly which has no sting but uses the biological language for 'beware I sting'.

(2)   Other forms of deception could develop within the lifetime of an individual and require more highly developed mental skills – genuine dishonesty.

(3)   But perhaps the most common form of apparent deception is a misunderstanding of honest signals.

In order for cheats to develop through natural selection, the benefit of the true signal to those who are deceived must outweigh the cost of being cheated at whatever rate the deception occurs. Otherwise selection will favour ignoring the signal.

The second requirement is that the cheats should not be found out. For example suppose the depth of the roar of a stallion is a sign of his fighting ability. There would be no advantage in being a small stallion with a deep roar. The deception just would not work.

Cheating behaviour strategies have been reported in other species. For example, a type of bird called the ringed plover will feign injury in order to lure a fox away from its nest when it has chicks (Slater, 1985). As long as it normally pays a fox to hunt apparently injured animals or for an alarm to mean alarm, there is no pressure for change in the species being duped. This form of deception does not apparently need to be learned from scratch by plovers and the behaviour could rather be instinctive.

A more complex form of deception is shown by another bird, the white–winged tanager shrike. If one of these birds is chasing a flying insect, it is likely to sound the alarm call, which says 'take cover, there's a hawk about' if another bird is also pursuing the insect. Many species of bird share similar alarm calls and so will take avoidance measures, even though there is no hawk about (Munn, 1986). The use of deceitful behaviour in this way implies some fairly sophisticated neural wiring in the brain but does not require either spitefulness or in fact any degree of consciousness.

In horses, honest signals may be used in a way that can easily be misunderstood. For example take the horse that threatens to kick but never does. Is the horse lying? Not necessarily. It could be an inhibited form of aggression, with the horse in a dilemma using its limited vocabulary to say 'I really want to get rid of this thing that is bugging me, but it's you and I really don't want to get rid of you'. If you persist he'll put up with it, because his attachment to you is stronger than his aversion to what you are doing. Alternatively it could be an old signal with a new meaning. It is normal for horses to use threats of aggression before they get physical. If someone is doing something to the horse which it does not like, the horse may issue an aggressive threat. This could be the horse's attempt at saying 'I don't like this, please stop, and if you persist I'll kick you'. In which case you will get kicked if you do not stop but, if you back off, the horse learns that this threat gets rid of people when they are doing something he dislikes. If this happens several times, the raised foot could be used more readily in any situation to signal 'leave me alone' even if it is not an actually an issue worth fighting about. When you keep going in these circumstances, you will not get kicked. It is not that he is lying and that you have called his bluff; it is just that he has learned a slightly new meaning to this act, which has broken free of its inevitable link to further aggression or running away.

It is important to recognise that some manipulative strategies are simply learned whilst others have a strong specific genetic foundation. Either way we should not be surprised that they occur, but we should resist the temptation to describe their motivation as having some form of emotional basis or moral quality, for example, by saying that the animal is being spiteful or mean. These comments only add confusion to the situation and do not help us in considering how to manage it any better. The extent to which horses manipulate the behaviour of others (including their owners) is not known.

Signals of communication

Perhaps some of the most notable behaviours displayed by horses, like rearing or prancing, are intentional signals. The fact that they are so striking maximises their clarity to the receiver but may also bring unwanted attention from potential predators. As with other issues in behaviour there is a trade off between the benefits and costs of any strategy, with the optimal strategy appearing as a result of natural selection on the variants.

It is perhaps not surprising therefore that when we look more closely we see a whole range of signals being used from the stylised and overt to the subtle. It is particularly the latter which tend to be missed or ignored and which lead to management problems. Signals may be intentional or otherwise but their interpretation depends on recognition of their structure.

Discrete or graded signals

Some signals are discrete (for example the presence or absence of an individual's scent on an object), whereas others are more obviously

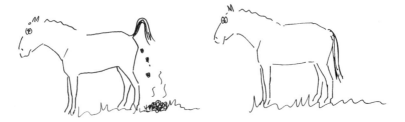

Fig. 7.2 Discrete signals are either there or not there, e.g. the appearance of a dung pile. Graded signals vary in their intensity, e.g. the scents associated with the dung vary with its age and the state of the depositor.

graded like the escalating series of threats used in defence encounters (see also Figure 7.6).

Simple and composite signals

They may be simple or composite. A composite signal has different meanings in different contexts. For example, Trumler (1958) reports that zebra mares in oestrus have a characteristic facial expression called 'rossigkeitsgesicht' which accompanies the normal wide-legged, tail to one side, stance. This is a composite signal of oestrus. The facial expression alone is not sufficient since without the accompanying body posture it is a threat of aggression.

Context

The context in which a signal is received may also affect its meaning. When a mare is in full oestrus a stallion will tend to ignore the urination of other females. If there are no mares in oestrus then a stallion often investigates all mares standing to urinate. Alternatively the timing of a signal in relation to others may affect its meaning. Horses often nip as an invitation to play and this behaviour signals that what follows, which may include threat gestures, is not a serious challenge. The use of a preliminary signal to define the meaning of those that follow in this way is called 'metacommunication'.

Medium

The medium used to transmit a deliberate signal is likely to be the one most appropriate to the type of message being transferred. Auditory, chemical, tactile and visual channels are all of great importance to the horse.

(1) **Auditory signals** can travel a long distance, allow a rapid exchange of information, and are not easily blocked by physical objects; but comparatively speaking they require a lot of energy to send. The signaller is also relatively easy to identify.

(2) **Chemical signals** also travel well but take longer to exchange and the sender is not necessarily so easy to identify. They are relatively cheap, energetically speaking, to send.

(3) **Tactile signals** obviously involve close contact for their transmission and are easily blocked by any physical obstacles. They do, however, allow for a rapid exchange and accurate identification of the signaller. They do not require as much energy to transmit as auditory signals and so are a low energy option.

(4) **Visual signals** travel a reasonable distance and can facilitate a very rapid exchange of information. The signaller is usually very obvious as they can be seen, but this view may easily be blocked by physical obstructions. Visual signals do not necessarily require a lot of effort depending on the nature of the signal.

Humans tend to consider the visual route first and think of the obvious visual displays that animals use in their communication, but this is not necessarily the most useful or most developed channel in other species. We should not be limited or biased by our own capacities.

Acoustic signals

In some species acoustic signals are beyond the range of human hearing and easily ignored. Whilst most horse sounds appear audible to the human ear, they may also contain significant inaudible elements (see Chapter 6).

(1) **Neighs and whinnies** signal an individual's presence. They tend to be used when a horse is separated or isolated from an associate, such as when a foal gets separated from its mother or an owner first appears on the yard and the horse is in a box. Since the noise may travel long distances, and indicates who the sender is and where they may be found, this is an obvious means of communication for such a message.

(2) **Nickers** appear to be a sign used to encourage an individual to come nearer. They are used by mares towards their foals, stallions when they wish to mate and by either sex towards approaching familiar people.

(3) **Squeals** are believed to be a defensive threat greeting used between highly aroused unfamiliar horses. They usually follow a nose to nose greeting and are often accompanied by a backward leap even though no bites have been exchanged. They may warn the recipient that more overt aggression will follow if provoked. They are often heard in response to acute pain such as when an injection is resented.

(4)　**Short snorts** are often heard when there is some degree of alarm, whereas a more prolonged sound is more usually associated with some form of frustration. Alarm snorts are also used in a play situation.

(5)　**Groans** are usually quite soft and often heard at times of

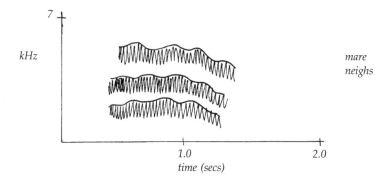

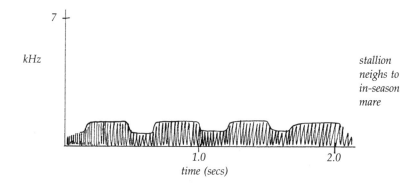

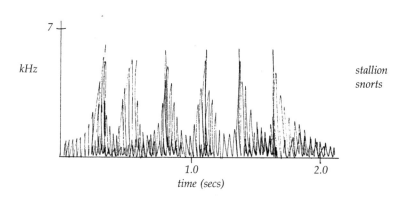

Fig. 7.3　Sonogram recordings of different auditory signals. Y-axis records frequency of sound.

discomfort or tiredness. They may also be heard occasionally from the horse confined for long periods in the stable.

(6)   **Roars and screams** are high intensity sounds made at times of extreme arousal. They seem to threaten severe physical violence, since they tend to be issued when more subtle signals have been ignored.

Most authors suggest that the calls communicate the level and type of arousal felt by the sender. But many owners claim to be able to discern more precise meanings from unspecified unique features associated with a particular call from their own horse. This may be the case, but equally it may reflect an owner's interpretation of a sound in a given context. Consistent subtle differences have not yet been demonstrated to show a more complex audible language.

Two other auditory signals include foot-stamping, which is usually a low level threat or sign of discomfort, and pawing, which may be a sign of frustration. The latter may become established as a repetitive and apparently functionless behaviour over time. It then joins behaviours like weaving, cribbing and stall-walking in a list of behaviour and welfare concerns known as stereotypies, which will be discussed in Chapter 10.

Chemical signals

The importance of chemical signals tends to be underestimated by man who, compared to most domestic species, has an extremely poor sense of smell. Chemicals do not have to be consciously detected for them to have an effect. Horses use both sniffing and the characteristic flehmen response in order to investigate social odours or pheromones. These are hormone-like chemicals released into the environment by an animal which affect the behaviour of other members of the same species.

Chemical signals are produced in skin secretions, saliva and possibly breath as well as the more obvious sources of urine and faeces. Equine greetings often involve olfactory investigation of the nose and mouth region, followed by the flanks and perineal regions. The latter appears to be particularly important in the identification of the foal, who, by shaking its tail as it feeds, wafts its odours towards the mare. This allows it to suckle without disturbance and certainly in the early stages of development may act as an important cue for the bonding process.

The role of cutaneous secretions in the horse is probably far more extensive than we currently realise. In other species, like the cat, some components have been shown specifically to inhibit inter- and intra-specific aggression and others appear to have a general calming effect.

As already discussed, a mare's urine signals her reproductive state, but once again there are undoubtedly other signals here as well. Tyler (1972) reports that young foals almost invariably urinated over their mother's urine marks. This behaviour does not extend into maturity when stallions cover only the urine of mares in oestrus.

Faeces probably act as both a visual and chemical signal. The recognition of familiar faeces may help in navigation and orientation, since Tyler also reports that mares which become separated from their group tend to sniff the faeces in the locality. Stallions also tend to defecate at particular sites along frequently used routes. This may help in orientation but also serves to declare his presence in an area. Stallions also cover the faeces of female members of the group whether or not they are in oestrus. It has been suggested that this repels intruders who may otherwise pursue a mare-only group. The association between elimination and communication helps to explain why a pasture will be more efficiently grazed by stallions than geldings or mares. The latter two are less discriminatory in their elimination but, like a stallion, will not normally graze near a dung pile and so larger areas of the pasture become unusable.

When a chemical produces a behaviour change such as the flehmen response or sexual arousal it is easy to recognise the importance of that chemical cue. This is not so obvious and is easier to ignore when the effect is more subtle, such as when it identifies an individual; all we may see after we have washed our horse is that he gets kicked or bitten by his normal companions. It is important to consider the importance of individual odour in such a situation and not to dismiss the possibility of our inadvertent involvement in the problem. If things are different after you do something then the chances are that what you have done has either directly or indirectly had an effect.

An even less obvious effect of chemical messengers involves their impact on growth and development. In other species it has shown that males are underweight and do not mature in the normal way if reared in same-sex groups. Simply introducing female urine into the areas where they are reared can rectify this.

Chemical signals may be involved in the following processes:
(1) Identification of the individual, including its sex, age and physiological state
(2) Co-ordinating and spacing individuals both within a social group and between different groups
(3) Mare–foal communication including bonding and the let down of milk
(4) Alarm and calm signalling
(5) Navigation and orientation

(6)   Sexual arousal and performance
(7)   Growth, development and maturity.

Tactile signals

Tactile signals used by horses range from those conveyed during grooming which have a de-arousing (calming) effect to those used in aggression like biting which cause excitement. At the inter-specific level we have similar goals when we stroke a familiar horse or using riding aids to encourage it to go faster in a race. Tactile signals are also used to direct an individual's behaviour whether that is a mother guiding her foal or a handler using a bit.

Grooming

Whilst horses are quite capable of grooming themselves, they tend to engage in bouts of mutual grooming when given the opportunity. Horses in small groups seem to groom every other individual in the group equally, but in larger groups clear favourites are often apparent. One horse will approach another with its ears forward, mouth slightly open and lower lip dropped to show the incisors. If the ears are laid back this may be an aggressive threat or signal a grooming approach from a more dominant individual. The two individuals then usually stand facing each other and nibble at their opposite number's neck, mane, forelegs and withers usually for about up to three minutes. Other regions of the body are involved less frequently and occasionally the behaviour occurs between three or more at the same time. In the vast majority of occasions these bouts are terminated by the dominant one of a pair. Tyler (1972) reports that foals will engage in what appears to be a version of this behaviour from day one.

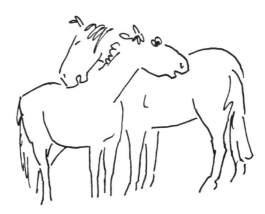

Fig. 7.4 Mutual grooming provides social tactile signals as well as parasite control.

The behaviour has a seasonal pattern, which corresponds with that of the annual moult and cycle of external parasites, but almost certainly it has a social function as well. It helps the members of a social group stay close and appears to be calming. Feh and de Mazieres (1993) showed that grooming of a preferred site reduces the heart rate of the horse compared to grooming of least preferred regions. The horse will usually respond to grooming of these preferred regions by gently extending its head, half closing its eyes and extending, gyrating and twitching its upper lip. This has been interpreted as a sign of intense pleasure by some (e.g. Waring 1983). In any case it is much easier to handle a horse which allows you to indulge in mutual grooming first.

Visual signals

As already discussed, horses have quite good vision. They are able to discriminate detail quite well and are particularly sensitive to movement within the visual field. It is not surprising therefore that these features play an important part in their visual signals.

Sudden or unusual movements are generally quite exciting to a horse, that is, they increase its arousal. Such movements are seen in a variety of threat displays such as the head threat (a sudden jerk forwards and up of the head), the foreleg strike and rearing as well as during the sexual displays of the stallion. This is combined with another common feature of visual signalling relating to the body outline; the relaxed horse has a long, extended posture, whereas the more excited animal is more gathered.

So how does one horse know how effectively he is getting another's attention? First there are general signs associated with the redirection of attention by a horse. When an animal notes that something different is going on in its environment, there is an

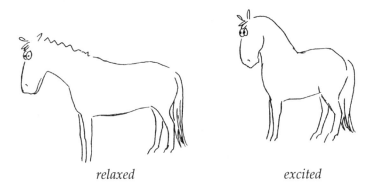

relaxed   *excited*

Fig. 7.5   Relaxed horses have a long extended outline, whilst excited horses are more rounded.

increase in arousal and the behavioural inhibition system comes into play (Gray, 1987). This causes all on-going activity to stop and starts to focus attention towards the cause of interest. One ear, two ears, the head or whole body may be turned towards the source. Once this has been investigated enough for it to be identified, an appropriate behavioural response may be made from one of the three options:

(1)   Flight, i.e. to run away
(2)   Fight, i.e. to stand your ground and defend yourself
(3)   Befriend, i.e. to stand your ground and try to defuse the situation by showing the required response.

Horses are not natural fighters but they will defend their position if they cannot escape or if they particularly value what they believe is being threatened. This is most often kin or a sexual partner. Tyler (1972) reports that mares, and Berger (1986) that stallions will occasionally intervene aggressively to assist an unrelated social companion to defend himself or herself. If a horse does decide to fight then we are likely to see an escalating series of threats, which will tend to go down one of two routes depending on the horse's assessment of the situation.

The normal submissive reaction from a horse is to calmly walk away, in order to avoid conflict. Occasionally it may do this with its ears held back (see Figure 7.6).

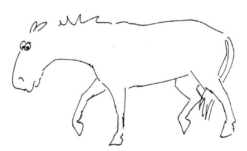

Fig. 7.6   Horse showing appeasement gesture.

But if a horse is not to run, there are a number of ways in which it may show appeasement in order to defuse the situation. It may throw its head up in the air but keep its attention on the one approaching. This way the whites of its eyes may be exposed. The tail is tucked between its hind-legs as it moves its hindquarters away. This suggests that the horse is mildly fearful but does not pose a threat unless these signs are ignored.

Unfortunately these initial signs being ignored is too often the case with a horse which has been disturbed in its stable. The horse may then issue non-physical threats of aggression, which may again be ignored until overt aggression is involved (see Figure 7.7). If this happens frequently, for example in a riding school with a large number of inexperienced handlers, the horse soon learns that these threats are ignored and overt aggression is the only signal that

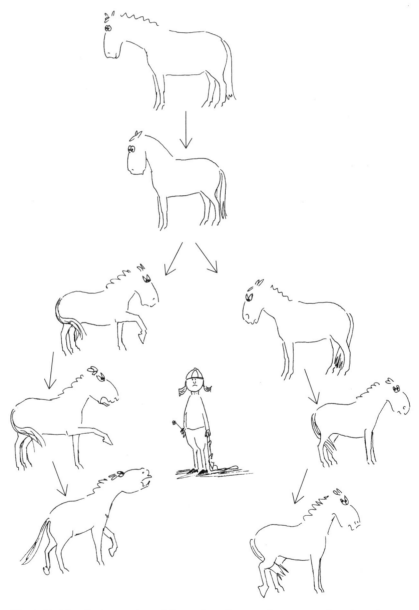

Fig. 7.7   Escalating series of frontal and posterior aggressive threats.

works. It therefore resorts to this behaviour at the first sign of disturbance and is soon labelled as a horse that bites for no apparent reason. Considering the history, however, tells us that there was good reason for the behaviour.

A more obvious cautious approach gesture is for the horse, with tucked tail, to lower its head, turn its ears outward and champ its teeth with its lips pulled back. The jaw movement (known as 'snapping' (Tyler, 1972) or 'Unterlegenheitsgebarde' (Zeeb, 1959)) is most commonly seen in younger horses, but may also be expressed by adults in certain situations. These tend to be when the animal has decided not to flee or try to dominate but would still appear to be uncertain about how its social deference will be received, for example just before 'join up' in the round pen technique, popularised by Monty Roberts (see Chapter 9). It is, in effect, testing a novel social situation. It would appear to be an indication of uncertainty in the approach or general anxiety and may therefore originate as a displacement behaviour (see Chapter 10).

The language of the horse is therefore a complex one of sights, sounds, smells and touches. If used correctly, it can help control and co-ordinate their behaviour without violence. Many signals have a natural meaning but we must be aware that learning and the stress of domestication can modify this.

Social organisation

Types of group

Horses are often considered to be a social species. That is, they tend to live in social groups. The structure and functioning of these groups falls under the realm of an area of science known as sociobiology. Groups of horses can be found together for two reasons.

Common focus (no cohesive bonds)

The first, is that they are brought together by some common focus such as the presence of a watering hole or a suitable river crossing. In this case the group is not a social unit, since individuals do not make an effort to stay together. That is, there are no cohesive bonds between the individuals. They may however engage in behaviours designed to keep them apart at this time, such as aggressive threat gestures. This form of equine group is occasionally seen in the wild for example Grevy's zebra (*Equus grevyi*) and Plains zebra (*Equus burchelli*) often come together in large single species or mixed species groups at water-holes within their overlapping ranges in Northern Kenya.

Social society (consistent relationships)

The second type of group is the social society in which most horses choose to live. These societies are defined by a consistent set of social relationships and interactions between members of the group. The animals make an effort to stay together. They engage in the three Cs of a stable social society:

◇ communication
◇ co-ordination
◇ cohesion.

For horses to live in such a society, they must be capable of the behaviours and mental activity required to hold a group (or band as it is known) together. This includes individual recognition, the co-ordination of activity and the performance of social exchanges to keep individuals close together.

Aggression is a sign that the relationships within a group are not fully established or not completely stable.

Social groups can be quite stable or transitory.

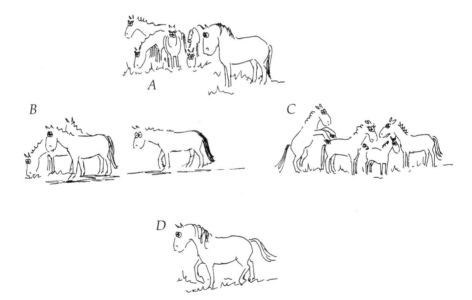

Fig. 7.8　Types of social organisation. A: stallion with harem B: bachelor band C: mixed sex non-breeding juvenile band D: lone stallion.

(1) **Stable social groups** These are groups in which the adults stay together for a number of years. Both family groups, in which one stallion lives with several mares and their young (harems) and all-male bachelor bands are recognised in free-ranging wild horses. Young, non-reproductively active

juveniles may break away or be driven out of the herd to form their own group, and adult stallions may also be found in isolation.

(2) **Transitory social groups** When Grevy's zebra migrate small social bands may join together to form much larger herds for the duration of the migration. These larger groups may themselves appear to coalesce into larger non-social groups at important environmental points such as river crossings or water-holes, as described above.

Why should a horse choose to live with others?

Living in a group has both advantages and disadvantages.

Advantages

(1) In a group there are a greater number of eyes looking out either for predators or food, and so a better chance of survival.

(2) If a predator does spot you and you are in a group, it may be possible to scare him off if you stick together alternatively, if you decide to run for it, there is a chance that in the chaos which follows that he will loose track of you.

(3) Groups are also more able to defend their resources better. It has been reported (Berger, 1986) that stallions who normally control a group of mares will, in certain circumstances, allow another stallion to join the band. It seems that this helps him fight off intruding males more effectively.

(4) Further advantages which might extend to the young, who represent the genetic future of the band's genes, include the occasional incidence of adoption and cross-fostering. Occasionally, a mare will allow a foal other than their own to suckle or a group adopts an unrelated foal in the absence of its mother (Blakeslee, 1974; Boyd, 1980).

Disadvantages

Set against these benefits, are the costs of group living.

(1) This includes the greater risk, to your offspring in particular, of being seriously injured and dying as a result of the behaviour of other members of the group, for example in a stampede or in competition over some resource.

(2) Competition over limited resources is more intense in a group, since, if you find something, so do all the other group members.

(3) Another potentially serious problem is the threat of infectious disease. If one of a group becomes infected then there is often a greater chance of others catching the same illness.

Overall we can conclude that if an individual chooses to live in a group then the benefits must outweigh the costs in the long term.

It is important to realise that groups tend to be adaptive in free management systems. There is no one social system which applies to all circumstances. Members of a social group adjust their behaviour, within their own limits, in order to stay together in the prevailing conditions.

What makes a band?

There have been many studies into the social organisation of horses. Some bands are all male, some of mixed sex and some, in man-made circumstances, all female, with the latter tending to be smaller than the breeding groups in similar situations (Tyler, 1972). In a variety of environments breeding groups of just a pair of individuals have been recorded (Feist & McCullough, 1975; Welsh, 1975; Green & Green, 1977; Greyling, 1994) but some groups in the same environment may contain more than 20 individuals (Feist & McCullough, 1975; Welsh, 1975). Average group sizes range from around three (Pellegrini, 1971) to more than twelve (Rubenstein, 1978) depending on the availablitlity of resources like food and water. Miller (1981), Berger (1986) and Greyling (1994) have all recorded breeding groups with two or more stallions and Ryden (1972) and Greyling (1994) have noted that some stallions only hold mares of a certain colour in their harems. In large open areas like Exmoor (Gates, 1979) and central Australia (Hoffmann, 1983) stallions do not attempt to defend territory against other males, whereas amongst dense island populations territorial behaviour has been recorded (Rubenstein, 1981).

What does this tell us about what is important in building a group? Some may suggest that it shows that the organisation of a group is random and of no real importance. To others it suggests that social groups are not just determined by the physical envir- onment but that a group exists because individuals make an effort to keep it together (the stallion in the case of a breeding group) and that these individuals have their own individual capabilities and preferences. We should be mindful of this complexity when con- sidering the groups that we want to keep in captivity, but first we need to know what factors to consider when we describe the group.

Not all groups are the same and, to understand a social group when we describe it, there are three key features that we need to consider:

◇ The composition of the group
◇ The social structure of the group
◇ The dynamics of the group.

The composition of the group

This describes its size and what individuals are in it, their age, sex, relatedness and any other individual characteristics that we can measure. We have already noted that horses do not naturally form social groups of more than about twenty. We have also said that in order to live in a proper social society individuals must be able to recognise others and remember their relationship with them. It may be therefore that twenty represents the mental limit of a horse's social memory. In which case we should be cautious about mixing more than about twenty horses together when space is quite limited. In fact, it is likely that a horse's social circle tends to be much smaller (less than ten). Beyond this they may not be able to organise themselves into a proper horse society and, if space is limited, they cannot divide themselves into sub-groups. As a result the horses appear to show a lot of aggression towards each other.

But what of the large herds that are seen in the New Forest, Camargue or Wyoming? These groups are more like a set of homes in a community. They may be together because of a common purpose and live together as a transitory social group because of the benefits of this. However each unit keeps itself separate. In this case we might like to think that a horse lives within a group of 'friends' with which it interacts positively. This group forms part of a larger community, consisting largely of strangers, with whom the horse is more cautious and from which it tends to keep its distance. This feature becomes apparent when we examine the second of the dimensions which describe a group.

The social structure of the group

This is determined by the type and quality of the relationships between individuals within the group. The relationships are themselves defined by the nature of the interactions seen to occur between members of the group (Hinde, 1976). The interactions between members or behaviours of an individual may also suggest that group members take up specific roles. This is where we will start with our description.

A stallion as group co-ordinator
Female groups tend to be larger if they include a stallion. Stallions with these groups spend time rounding up females and stopping them from dropping out of the group. They herd and drive the group (see Figure 8.5). We could therefore say that one of the roles of the stallion is to encourage the group to stay together. When the

harem moves, the stallion tends to be the last in the group and this may again be associated with his role as a group co-ordinator.

A mare as group leader

In many groups the oldest mare will go in front. The most logical reason for this consistent trend is that the oldest mare has probably travelled the route more than any other mare and so is more familiar with the terrain and its potential hazards. It is therefore adaptive and advantageous to allow elders to go first, to be the group leader.

A controller of an activity

By watching groups of horses we can identify other roles, for example the movement or action of one individual may lead to the rest of the group doing the same. This animal may then be described as the controller of this activity. The effectiveness of a controller depends on the individual horse and what it is trying to control.

Socially facilitated behaviour

When behaviour is more likely to occur when someone else is doing it, it is said to be socially facilitated. This is an important co-ordinating and cohesive force within a group. In horses it tends to apply to behaviours like grazing, resting, shelter seeking and, most importantly, running away. The relationship between individuals may affect the power of this force. It is stronger between individuals who are more closely associated or between those already in a similar motivational state when one starts the behaviour. Sometimes one individual initiates an activity but the group, as a whole, does not follow unless or until a specific individual (the controller) joins in. The controller in these circumstances may then be described as a dominant individual. This sophisticated but beautiful process is well illustrated in Tyler's records (1972) of New Forest Pony behaviour. She records how certain individuals could initiate a move to a new location but, having started the process, they would stand and wait until another individual took the lead.

Dominance or control?

There is often a lot of confusion over the role of dominance in the control of equine behaviour. Dominance is apparent when one individual controls the behaviour of another or controls access to some resource. It is a product of the interactions between two or more individuals and is most often recognised as a result of aggressive encounters. In this situation you will usually have a winner and a loser. The winner is dominant to the subordinate loser. When an individual consistently wins or loses encounters with another we can assign them a rank. One can say that the winner ranks more highly and so has an earlier (smaller) number. If we consider all the competitive encounters within a group of say eight, then we may be able to assign ranks one to eight to each individual according to who they can dominate. Number one, the alpha individual, can control everyone and number eight, the omega individual, has control over no one. This is known as a dominance hierarchy.

A general social hierarchy relates to all competitive encounters, and we should not propose a social hierarchy on the basis of one particular type of competition, e.g. competition over food. A specific hierarchy may tell us the importance of controlling a particular activity or resource to each individual within the group during a given observation period.

A common problem extending from the idea of dominance is: the emphasis it puts on the ability of a single individual to gain overall control of everything. It is possible to construct a general hierarchy for a group of horses but it will not be as simple as the one described above. We are most unlikely to find a single individual always winning every encounter if different individuals have different roles. Even if we just use the trend in the relationship, triangular relationships become apparent. These structures may seem nice, but their importance to the horses living in the group is questionable.

A further complication is the importance of group dependent relationships, that is the presence of a close associate of the subordinate on the outcome of an encounter. To date most studies of equine social behaviour have ignored this possibility although it is well recognised that individual horses have allies with whom they prefer to spend time. Individuals have also been reported to intervene on behalf of each other, a factor that cannot be easily illustrated in the sort of data table described above.

Aggression
Horses in a social group co-operate in order to avoid aggression whenever possible for a number of reasons:

(1)   Aggression takes a lot of energy which could be used for other functions
(2)   Aggression involves serious risks to your health and fitness
(3)   Aggression separates individuals and so does not strengthen the grouping tendency.

Social aggression is a sign of some uncertainty about the relationship between two individuals. When this is well established, the subordinate will tend to avoid the dominant individual or defer to him when either approaches the other. When horses do use aggression, they use a series of escalating threats (see Figure 7.7) before they resort to physical violence. This is for the reasons described above.

The flight zone

There is more to social bonding, however, than the avoidance of violent competition. Social partners allow each another to get closer when there is no competition. At this time they also engage in close mutual exchanges, like grooming (see Figure 7.4). Social partners, or friends for want of a better phrase, are tolerated within an individual's normal 'flight zone' and even allowed access to its 'personal space'.

The flight zone is the space around a horse, which, if entered, will cause it to move away. It varies from individual to individual and from situation to situation. It tends to be greater in more timid horses or when a horse is very excited.

The personal space is the area immediately around a horse in which only close companions are tolerated. If, having ignored more subtle aggressive signals, you cross over this line when you are not welcome, it is normal for a horse to respond violently as this is his final defence, although some will show an uncomfortable acceptance. For the sake of our horse's well-being we want to make sure we are welcome rather than timidly tolerated in this area.

We will discuss how we can exploit these zones for humane management and training later (see Chapter 9), but a general reduction and inhibition of aggression at several levels is an important way in which we can recognise and build affiliation and friendship.

The results of captivity

Aggression between horses is more often seen in captivity than in the wild for several reasons, not least because:

(1) Space is more limited and so competition for resources may be more intense
(2) Limited space means that there is less opportunity for a submissive horse to retreat far enough
(3) Forced confinement leads to horses inadvertently entering the personal space of others when they are not welcome
(4) By constantly taking horses in and out of the group, even for short periods of time, we risk upsetting the established social structure.

Training using social bonds

The evolution of horses suggests that they will respond better to control based on non-violent leadership and instruction. In the wild, this tends to come from the signs and signals of other horses and learned associations (see above). In the domestic situation we want horses to respond to us. For really effective training, then, we need to be aware of the natural signals which we can communicate to the horse like 'beware', 'relax', 'stop' and 'move on', but also we must teach the horse many new responses.

As with socially facilitated behaviour (see above), our relationship with our horse will affect the ease with which this information is communicated. A horse which is 'dominated' by violence and punishment techniques is fearful and not in an optimal state to learn. A horse with which we form a close mutual bond is in a better state to respond to our requests because of its natural tendency to co-operate with social partners. This relationship is illustrated both in trying to spend time together and in sharing socially important activities like mutual grooming. When training it is important to use a language your horse can understand to establish a position of control rather than dominance.

The dynamics of the group

This is the rate of change around the group; the length of time it has been together and the rates at which individuals join or leave it. Strong individual relationships may last a lifetime and so we should consider carefully the effect of management systems that break up groups on a periodic basis. It seems that sometimes when we remove an individual from a group, the group reorganises. New affiliations and alliances are made and new roles adopted. As a result, when we try to reintroduce the original horse, he may no longer recognise the social structure of the group. This sort of instability may then cause considerable aggression as the individual tries to establish or recognise a new organisation.

It is normal for colts and fillies to leave their mother's band any time after the first year. Colts may leave voluntarily or be forced out by the resident stallion. Fillies are more readily tolerated and may stay within the group, in which case they appear to maintain a close association with their mothers and can frequently be seen to indulge in mutual grooming. Weaning and dispersal are normally gradual processes in the wild but often rapidly enforced in captivity. It is now thought that these dynamic changes and the stress they cause may predispose horses to a number of behavioural problems, including stereotypic behaviours. We will discuss these problems in the chapter on welfare.

Juveniles are not the only ones to move between groups. The stallion usually moves behind the group to make sure that none get left behind, but a heavily pregnant mare will often get left behind when she is about to foal. This seems to be one time when she may be picked up by another stallion. Contrary to popular belief such a stallion tends not to kill the new-born foal.

The other important time of change comes as a result of a challenge from another stallion. A resident stallion may try to prevent these threats either by controlling access to the area in which the group lives (territorial defence) or by defending the mares more specifically and wherever they may be (dominance type system). A number of signals are used to keep males apart and to avoid unnecessary conflict. Once deposed the former resident will not normally get another chance to breed.

The mares represent the future prospects for the resident stallion's genes and so he can be expected to defend them at great personal expense against invaders. When considering the defence of the group many of the principles that apply to control by individuals apply at the higher level of groups. Whereas an individual horse may have a reaction distance of about four metres, within which it will react to defend itself, for groups it tends to be 50 metres or more. This is the distance that groups tend to try and keep between each other. One group may dominate another and, if they arrive in the same area, the subordinate group will move on or may wait for the others to pass through. Any nearer and the resident stallions can be expected to become defensive.

How horses defend their resources

The home range
The area normally covered by a band of horses is known as its home range. These will often overlap with other bands and can vary in size from whatever area we allow in captivity to more than 50 square kilometres (Green & Green, 1977). The size of the home range does not depend on the size of the group as much as it does on the shape and nature of the land. In some wild areas of land it may be as little as 3 square kilometres (Rubenstein, 1981).

Stud piles and marking
Within the home range the stallion will mark over the eliminations of the females and leave specific dung piles (stud piles). Mares on the other hand have a very different response to faeces. If a mare sees another mare defecate then she is likely to do the same (we might say that defecation is a socially facilitated behaviour in mares). However if she comes across the dung of another mare but has not seen it produced she is more likely to urinate over it after

sniffing it. It is thought that the freshness of these marks might indicate how close another group is and helps to keep the groups apart. The stallion's mark over a mare's tells any outsider that she is already taken. If a mare gets separated from her harem she is more likely to sniff any eliminations which she encounters, probably in order to try a follow the trail back.

The core area

Within the home range there is often a core area in which most activity is concentrated. This is less likely to overlap between groups and includes preferred sites for grazing, shelter, drinking and shade. In the domestic environment we do not normally allow for these. This may lead to increased aggression between individuals as groups are forced to share facilities in a common core area.

Territoriality

Whilst horses seem to have preferred areas, they do not generally defend complete territories in the wild. Land outside the core area is occupied more on a time-share basis. Rubenstein (1981) reports that some harems on Shackleford Banks would defend territories. This is an exceptional situation as other reports suggest that individuals are guarded rather than areas. This behaviour may be a result of the peculiar geography of the area. Along some narrow lengths of the island the land is open, provides all the essential herbage and allows good visibility. In these circumstances it is suggested that it is more effective to defend a patch rather than guard a ranging group of females. Territorial behaviour is also distinguished by the use of clear dung signals at the periphery which tell others to keep out.

   The horse no doubt has the potential to operate a variety of social systems, depending on the environment. Whilst rare in the wild, the sort of conditions which encourage territoriality may be more common in the domestic situation as the areas given over to horses are generally very much smaller, but open and well resourced. Since the strategies used by a horse tend to be those that are best adapted to the prevailing conditions, the behaviour may occur more frequently than we realise. It is therefore worth considering this possibility in some cases of persistent domestic conflict.

Dominance

The more normal situation in the wild is control based on dominance. In this situation the stallion controls access to the harem because of who he is rather than where he is. In effect he says 'I don't care where I am; these are my mares, so keep away from them. And if you dare to come near I'll show you exactly who I am.' In the territorial system described above, he says, 'This is my patch, so keep off!' If any male ignores these messages he is greeted at close quarters with a tensely muscled strident snorting display. If this does not suitably intimidate him, then each may size the other up and release a pile of dung. They may squeal and roar at each other, threaten and try to drive one another away before they come to blows. Winner takes all.

This is a high risk game to play, and unless the intruder is confident of his position then he is likely to be seriously injured even if he wins. In which case he cannot defend his prize against another and the effort will be wasted. This is why posturing ritual and the avoidance of real violence is so important in nature.

The animals do not have to be able to know what the consequences of their actions are, in order to respond appropriately, they just have to be able to read and respond to the signs and act accordingly. Whilst the stallion is concerned with dominating any potential rivals, his marking displays over the eliminations of mares are more like the behaviour of a possessive territorial animal. Perhaps the best way to interpret this is that the harem is a mobile territory and what the stallion is trying to say to the world is 'These are mine so watch out!'

Conclusion

In order to manage horses effectively and sympathetically it is important to communicate with them in a way that they can understand. Possession seems important to stallions with mares, but bachelor bands will only try to take possession when they are clearly at an advantage. Mares are more dependent on affiliation for their loyalty, although males are also capable of forming strong ties. Good management should try to help people to form a close bond with their horses whilst maintaining the role of controller. This should avoid conflict and produce animals that are obedient because they want to respond favourably rather than ones that obey because they are scared to disobey.

Remember the building blocks of an effective partnership are effective:

◇ communication
◇ co-ordination and
◇ cohesion.

TOPICS FOR DISCUSSION

◇ Compare and contrast the advantages and disadvantages of the visual, auditory and chemical channels for communicating certain types of message.

◇ Consider in what situations a person might deliver conflicting signals to a horse through different channels.

◇ Discuss the similarities and differences between human and equine intra-specific communication.

◇ Discuss how you could conduct a study into the function or meaning of a certain horse signal.

◇ Discuss why some horses might appear to be anti-social.

◇ Design a study to investigate how the social behaviour of horses changes with increasing space allowance. What changes might you expect in their behaviour?

◇ Should we abandon the term 'dominance' when talking about equine social systems?

◇ How do the three key features of a wild horse social group (composition, social structure and dynamics) differ from those of a typical domestic one? What problems might arise from this?

References and further reading

Berger, J. (1986) *Wild Horses of the Great Basin*. University of Chicago Press, Chicago.

Blakeslee, J.K. (1974) *Mother–young relationships and related behaviour among free ranging Appaloosa horses*. MS Thesis, Idaho State University.

Boyd, L. E. (1980) *The natality, foal survivorship and mare–foal behaviour of feral horses in Wyoming's Red Desert*. MS Thesis, University of Wyoming.

Feh, C. & de Mazières, J. (1993) Grooming at a preferred site reduces heart rate in horses. *Animal Behaviour* **46**, 1191–4.

Feist, J.D. & McCullough, D.R. (1975) Reproduction in feral horses. *Journal of Reproduction and Fertility, (Supplement)* **23**, 13–18.

Feist, J.D. & McCullough, D.R. (1976) Behavior patterns and communication in feral horses. *Zeitschrift fur Tierpsychologie* **41**, 337–71.

Gates, S. (1979) A study of the home ranges of free-ranging Exmoor ponies. *Mammal Review* **9**, 3–18.

Gray, J.A. (1987) *The Psychology of Fear and Stress*. 2nd edn Cambridge University Press, Cambridge.

Green,N.F. & Green, H.D. (1977) The wild horse population of Stone Cabin Valley, Nevada: A preliminary report. In: *Proceedings of The National Wild Horse Forum*, R–127, 59–65 University of Nevada.

Greyling, T. (1994) *The behavioural ecology of the feral horses in the Namib Naukluft Park*. MSc Thesis, University of Pretoria.

Hinde, R.A. (1976) Interactions, relationships and social structure. *Man* **11**, 1–17.

Hoffmann, R. (1983) Social organisation patterns of several feral horse and feral ass populations in Central Australia. *Zeitschrift fur Saugetierkunde* **48**, 124–6.

Miller, R. (1981) Male aggression, dominance and breeding behavior in Red Desert feral horses. *Zeitschrift fur Tierpsychologie* **57**, 340–51.

Munn, C.A. (1986) Birds that 'cry wolf'. *Nature* **319**, 143–5.

Pellegrini, S.W. (1971) *Home range, territoriality and movement patterns of wild horses in the Wassuk range of western Nevada.* MS Thesis, University of Nevada.

Rubenstein, D.I. (1981) Behavioural ecology of island feral horses. *Equine Veterinary Journal* **13**, 27–34.

Ryden, H. (1972) *Wild Horses.* Secker & Warburg, London.

Slater, P.J.B. (1985) *An Introduction to Ethology.* Cambridge University Press, Cambridge.

Trumler, E. (1959) Das 'Rossigtkeitsgesicht' und ahnliches Ausdrucks-verhalten bei Einhufern. *Zeitschrifdt fur Tierpsychologie* **16**, 478–88.

Tyler, S. J. (1972) The behaviour and social organisation of the New Forest ponies. *Animal Behaviour Monographs* **5** (2).

Waring, G.H. (1983) *Horse Behavior: The Behavioural Traits and Adaptations of Domestic and Wild Horses, including Ponies.* Noyes, Park Ridge.

Welsh, D.A. (1975) *Population, behavioural and grazing ecology of the horses of Sable island, Nova Scotia.* PhD Thesis, Dalhousie University.

Wilson, E.O. (1976) *Sociobiology: The New Synthesis.* Harvard University Press, Harvard.

Zeeb, K. (1959) Verhaltensforschung beim Pferd. *Tierarztliche Umschau* **14**, 334–41.

8. Sexual and Reproductive Behaviour of Horses

We have already seen that there are several different types of social group in which horses can live, including groups in which a reproductively active male is a normal permanent feature of the unit. Other hoofed mammals (ungulates) tend not to adopt this strategy. This may explain, in part, the numerous other unique sexual behavioural characteristics of the horse, which must be considered when attempting to manage this species successfully in the domestic environment. For example, mares have a longer oestrus than most other ungulates (up to around 10 days may be normal, although 3–5 days is often considered typical) and it is has been suggested (Kiley-Worthington, 1987) that this may be important in establishing the necessary bond between the sexes. During this time the mare and stallion spend a considerable amount of time signalling to each other.

There are inevitable changes which can be expected as a result of domestication (see Chapter 3) and more recent selection, but we still do not fully understand the normal underlying physiology. The likely importance of social and individual factors only muddies the waters further. Horses have many special and unique features to their sexuality and whilst generalisations are possible (and necessary), perhaps one of the most striking features of this species is the range of individual variability in their reproductive behaviour.

This chapter will consider the factors which, together, mould the sexual behaviour of the horse. The management of the domestic horse, especially value animals like Thoroughbreds, is so radically different to the natural state that it is not surprising that breeding success is reportedly so poor. In some Thoroughbred studs, 70% of mares conceive and 50% produce a live foal, for mares in a wild harem the figure is believed to be around 95%.

Basic genetic foundation of the individual's sexuality

This establishes whether an individual is a male or female horse. There are two components to consider here.

(1)   Firstly, that the individual is a horse and so will develop the specific traits of horses rather than any other species.
(2)   Secondly that the individual will develop a set of gonads associated with a specific sex, i.e. testes or ovaries. These are responsible for the release of sexual hormones which affect development before birth and at puberty. Oestrogens and androgens are responsible for the activation of sexual behaviour in female and male horses respectively at maturity. This is not a dose-dependent but an all-or-nothing response, i.e. if there is sufficient hormone the behaviours will develop but if there is excess this will not make the behaviour stronger. Once the gonads have developed, the genetic make-up of the individual is actually of little significance in the control and development of sexual behaviour.

The genes set in motion the physical framework for the normal pattern of sexual behaviour. This represents the basic ethology of reproductive behaviour in horses and will be considered first. To this we will add consideration of the acquired traits and more subtle genetic effects, which help account for the enormous variations seen. Perhaps in no other behaviour category are the differences of individuals so apparent.

Normal mare specific behaviour

This consists of the behaviours associated with the attraction and acceptance of a stallion, the behaviours of pregnancy and parturition, and maternal behaviour.

Attraction and acceptance of the stallion

The breeding season
Mares which do not become pregnant will have several sexual cycles within a specific period during the year. That is to say they are seasonally polyoestrous, with each oestrous cycle normally lasting around 21 days. The start and end of the breeding season are not fixed but regulated by changes in day length and so vary around the world. The season often starts soon after the spring equinox (i.e. the time in spring when the lengthening day equals the shortening night) and usually finishes soon after the autumnal equinox. The transition into and from the period of sexual inactivity is gradual. During this time, mares may show extended, partial or weak oestral behaviour. Early in the season they may produce but not fully mature the egg-bearing follicles, which control several aspects of the behaviour of the oestrous cycle, whilst at the other end of the season it appears to take longer for follicles to become activated.

The start of the season is initiated because information relating to changes in day length coming through the eyes is relayed to the pineal gland in the brain where it triggers a chain of chemical signals, which ultimately affect the ovary. The change in day length affects the pattern of release of melatonin from the pineal gland. This change then results in an alteration in the production of the releasing hormones (gonadotrophin releasing factors) from the hypothalamus.

The sexual cycle

Gonadotrophin releasing factors control the level of gonadotrophins in the blood. Specifically this group of chemicals consists of follicle stimulating hormone and luteinising hormone. The former cause the egg-bearing follicles to develop within the ovary whilst the latter bring about their release. As the follicles develop within the ovary they produce the oestrogens which bring about the behavioural changes of oestrus. The gonadotrophins are the essential link between the brain and the rest of the body for the physiological and behavioural aspects of the sexual cycle.

Under the influence of luteinising hormones the follicle ruptures to release the egg and transforms into a more solid yellow body

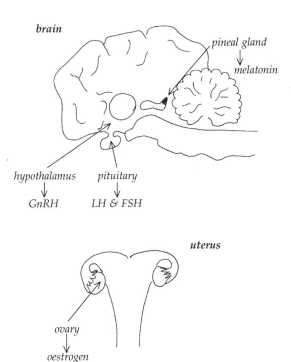

Fig. 8.1   Schematic diagram of the main endocrine organs involved in the sexual cycle of the mare.

(corpus luteum) which produces the hormone progesterone. In about a quarter of cycles more than one follicle develops and more than one egg is shed. Whilst each of these may be fertilised it is uncommon for both to survive. Only about one in a hundred foalings are twin births (Stabenfeldt & Edqvist, 1984), and most cases where twin foetuses start to develop result in spontaneous abortion around nine months.

The timing of ovulation affects the time spent in oestrus (heat) and this is usually around five or six days. If it is delayed for any reason then oestrus will be extended but there should still be 15–16 days between heats. If a pregnancy is not established the corpus luteum degenerates and this allows new follicles to mature. In as many as one in five cases the corpus luteum may persist beyond this time and delay the onset of the next cycle (Stabenfeldt & Edqvist, 1984). In many cases the cause of this remains unknown although in some chronic changes in the uterus are involved. During the acute phase of any disease of the womb the corpus luteum is more likely to break down sooner rather than later and cycles are shortened.

The breeding cycle

Females usually show their first heat as yearlings but do not appear to be as attractive to stallions at this age. After foaling the first period of full oestrus occurs around a week later and then every 21 days until the mare conceives. Under natural conditions mares will most often conceive during one of the first two cycles after foaling. Since the pregnancy lasts about 11 months mares will tend to give birth every 12 months. A mare is rarely barren. The advantage of coming into season in the spring is clear. Foals are most likely to be born when environmental conditions are improving.

From an evolutionary point of view, those mares which were not seasonal breeders would deliver foals at less favourable times of year and they would be less likely to survive. They therefore left fewer offspring than those which happened to be seasonal breeders and so had fewer representatives in the next generation. This trend continued until the only viable breeding population was that with the most efficient breeding pattern.

Whilst these pressures may no longer exist in captivity, there is no pressure for the system to be otherwise and so the trait can be expected to remain, albeit in a less rigid form. This applies even to Thoroughbreds which have their official birthday on 1 January and where much effort is made to breed them early. There is no selective pressure for earlier breeding in these circumstances because the individuals are themselves normally seasonally poly-oestrus and the techniques used to bring the mares into season earlier (like extended lighting or hormone treatments) do not have a genetic basis which can be passed from one generation to another.

Reproductive behaviours

When sexually cycling, periods of oestrus are separated by quite abrupt and distinctive 15–16 day periods of dioestrus when the mare shows no interest in the stallion. This should not be confused with the period of anoestrus which occurs between seasons and when she is equally uninterested in the stallion. Different physiological states exist at these two times.

Three distinct types of behaviour during oestrus, which can occur in the presence of a stallion, may help indicate a mare's reproductive state.

(1)   **The level of attraction** Individuals show mutual attraction by tolerating close contact with each other in their personal space (see Chapter 7) and exchanging social care-giving behaviour, like mutual grooming. The mare also attracts the attention of the stallion with a characteristic 'saw-horse' stance, which appears identical to that used at the time of copulation. She lowers her head, lays her ears back and out to the side, relaxes the face, straddles her hind legs, lowers her pelvis, and frequently passes small amounts of urine; this is then followed by repeated abdominal tensing which rhythmically expose her clitoris. This 'clitoral winking', as it is known, may also occur at other times during the oestrus period. It is more readily visible in horses since they tend to hold their tails to one side as they do it, ponies on the other hand tend more often to hold their tail straight back and half raised as they wink. It is thought that this behaviour helps in the spread of a chemical attractant (pheromone) from the tissues of the region.

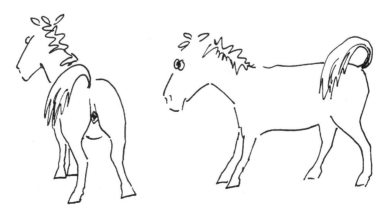

Fig. 8.2   Typical mare stance during oestrus. Rear and side views.

(2)   **The amount of proceptive behaviour**   At this time the mare and stallion appear actively to seek one another out. Mares may seek the stallion and position themselves in his way. Older and more dominant mares may actively interrupt the attention that a stallion is giving to a lower ranking female in oestrus. The proceptive behaviour of a particular mare towards a male horse used to detect when she is in oestrus (a teaser) may also mask the signals of other receptive mares. So teasing should be done on a one to one basis.

(3)   **The level of receptivity**   This is gauged from the extent to which a mare allows copulation to occur. The mare stands calmly as described above in order to accept the mounting stallion. A description of the normal copulatory process is given in the section on stallion behaviour.

These signs have been reported to occur spontaneously and occasionally in anoestrus mares (Waring, 1983; Asa, 1986). This has led to the suggestion that sexual behaviour may serve to reinforce the social bond between individuals of the same social group. However, the mature wild mare is normally pregnant for eleven months of the year, and so it is difficult to argue how or why such a system would have evolved.

Domestic breeding situations often place great emphasis on the first and last of these acts for the determination of the right time for breeding. Often, management practices do not allow the mare to seek out the stallion but the stallion is brought to the mare. The use of a stallion teaser to demonstrate attraction is relied on as a sign of receptivity but allowing proceptive behaviour may be important in ensuring a successful pregnancy or future receptivity.

The dioestral mare shows no great interest in males and, if approached by a courting stallion, she may be aggressive, flattening her ears back, screaming, biting, striking with her front legs and kicking with her hind legs. However, inhibited aggression is sometimes seen in the courting behaviour of some mares in oestrus and may easily be mistaken for dioestral behaviour. Superimposed on this structure are the individual characteristics and preferences of the mare or stallion. For example, the nervous mare may be aggressive to the stallion in a way that is similar to when she is in dioestrus; mares occasionally or habitually show no overt behavioural signs of oestrus (silent heats) even though their circulating hormone levels are normal and they are fully receptive. This has been estimated to occur in 7% of cases (Waring, 1983) and would suggest that the problem lies centrally within the parts of the brain controlling the overt behavioural signs of oestrus. This tends to suggest that external factors play a very large part in shaping the normal cyclical behaviour of the mare. These will be discussed in more detail below.

The complexity of the sexual cycle in the mare, including the absence of signs when a stallion is not in the area, can make the detection of oestrus by man quite difficult. Marthe Kiley-Worthington (1987) has suggested that training a dog to detect and signal the presence of the pheromones released by the receptive female may offer a practical solution to many of these difficulties.

Pregnancy and parturition

Pregnancy

Pregnancy in the mare usually lasts around 330–345 days. Slightly longer gestation periods tend to occur in mares carrying colt foals (Stabenfeldt & Edqvist, 1984), in the larger breeds (Fraser, 1992) and less well-fed mares (Hintz, 1977). If an egg has been fertilised, it signals its presence by affecting oestrogen levels within the mare by the fourteenth day post-fertilisation. This interferes with the otherwise inevitable degeneration of the corpus luteum, changes the pattern of production of further eggs and leads to the termination of the behavioural signs of the sexual cycle.

High levels of progesterone and lower levels of oestrogen are important in maintaining pregnancy. Unlike other domestic animals, the progesterone needed to maintain pregnancy is not freely detectable in the general circulation, but concentrated locally in the placenta. This may explain a common but unusual phenomenon often seen in pregnant mares. It has been estimated that as many as one in ten mares may show some of the signs of oestrus when they are pregnant (Satoh & Hoshi, 1933). These are usually proceptive behaviours. It is believed that this occurs more frequently if the mare is producing a lower level of progesterone. It is most commonly seen between the sixth and tenth weeks of pregnancy when it is normal for a second crop of follicles to develop into corpora lutea which by producing progesterone help maintain the pregnancy. The mare does not normally demonstrate receptive behaviour at this time. Whilst pregnant, mares tend to stay with their normal social group and engage in the normal range of social behaviours although they may have a preference for company of other pregnant mares.

Parturition triggers and timing

Parturition is triggered by a reversal of the ratio of oestrogen to progesterone hormone levels. Whilst levels of the former rise, progesterone levels fall. This is the result of changes in the metabolism of both the foetal foal and its mother. Nonetheless, mares seem to have an incredible amount of control over the timing of foaling. This may have served the modern horse's ancestors well since it allowed the mare to give birth when there was little risk of either mother or foal or both being eaten. It is reported that 80% of foalings occur at night (Fraser, 1992). Such a tendency gives the newborn foal longer to get to its feet and co-ordinate itself so that it can move with the grazing herd in the daylight. Parturition is also often very quick when it does take place and may be over in a matter of a few minutes.

The parturition process
The normal sequence of events is described below.

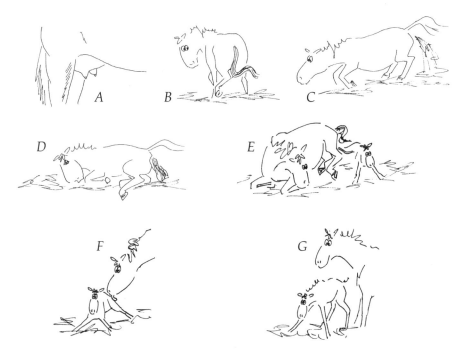

Fig. 8.3 Stages of parturition: (A) Waxing up of enlarged udder. (B) First stage labour. (C) Water breaking. (D) Parturition. (E) Post partum pause. (F) Maternal licking. (G) Foal standing and delivery of the placenta.

(A) **Preparation for parturition**
　　◇ 3–4 weeks before parturition the mare's udder is noticeably enlarged.
　　◇ A few days before the birth small beads of wax may appear at the ends of the teats (waxing up) and fluid may be seen to gather under the skin.

(B) **Immediately before birth – first stage labour**
◇ The mare keeps switching between behaviours and wanders around aimlessly (appears restless).
◇ Tail swishing, head turning towards flanks, kicking at belly, pawing at bedding, crouching, and frequent urination may all occur.
◇ The mare may lie down and stand up again shortly afterwards.
◇ Patches of sweat appear on the mare's flanks.
This phase may last minutes or hours. Alternatively it may start and then stop before resuming several hours or even days later.

(C) **Water breaking**
Bursting of the waters is often followed by a flehmen reaction to the uterine fluids and possible nicker calls.

(D) **Parturition – second stage labour**
◇ The mare lies down on her side, often with her uppermost hind leg extended.
◇ She strains forcefully and regularly to deliver the foal, but is usually able to interrupt the straining if disturbed.
◇ The mare may rest between bouts of contractions and even feed at this time.
◇ Straining usually lasts 10–30 minutes until the main trunk of the foal is delivered.
◇ The foal's movements rupture the surrounding sac and it pulls its own hind legs away from its mother.

(E) **Post partum pause**
The mare should remain lying for 15–20 minutes, but 25% in captivity stand within five minutes snapping the cord early. During this time blood passes from the mare to the foal and whilst the blood vessels in the cord may appear to be actively pumping blood into the foal, the volume of blood involved in transfer is believed to be quite small and the significance of this has been questioned (Doarn *et al.* 1987).

(F) **Maternal licking**
Mare licks foal and usually nickers. This marks the onset of the mare–foal bond and normal maternal behaviour.

(G) **Foal standing and delivery of the placenta**
◇ The foal, encouraged by the mare normally stands within an hour of the onset of licking and can walk within an hour of standing.
◇ The placenta is normally expelled within about two hours of the delivery of the foal, but many will complete this within an hour.
◇ Mares do not normally eat their placenta but walk away from it.

Robert Miller suggests that imprint training (see Chapter 4) should start at this time but this depends on having a mare who will accept people at this time and suitably skilled personnel who do not upset the development of the mare–foal bond. It needs to be borne in mind that previous temperament is not necessarily a good guide to a mare's behaviour at this time. A normally placid and friendly individual may become quite excitable or aggressive.

Normal maternal behaviour

Suckling

Soon after the foal rises the mare usually stands to allow it to suckle. She may turn to guide the foal towards the teat and will normally allow it to suckle for up to 20 minutes. The foal learns to suckle as described earlier in Chapter 4. Within the first three hours or so the foal will normally suckle again and pass the foetal faecal plug (meconium). The foal will feed almost hourly for the first day or so and the mare moves from licking to sniffing the foal at this time. When the mare ends the nursing bouts she does so by shifting her weight from one hind limb to the other before simply walking away from the suckling foal. Any aggression shown at this time is usually a response to the foal's over-zealous attempts to suckle and stimulate milk let down by banging her udder with its head.

Keeping contact

The mare and foal will normally move away from the foaling site and placenta soon after the first feed. The foal stays close to its mother, i.e. within about five metres (Tyler, 1972) for virtually the whole of the first week and is allowed to suckle at will. During this time the foal actively tries to stay near its mother when it is awake and it tends to be the mare which instigates any separation. It is thought that by leaving the foal and causing it to follow, the mare encourages imprinting and social bonding by the foal. However, when the foal is asleep the mare takes up the responsibility for maintaining close contact by grazing around the sleeping animal. The mare will rejoin and participate in the normal activities of her social group during the first week. At first she will block the foal from receiving attention from other horses in the group. After the first few days, however, the closest companions of the mare, including relatives, are allowed access to the foal. If the mare still has a yearling at foot this individual will follow behind the pair as the group moves on. The mare will normally start the sexual cycle again within ten days of the birth of the foal and may conceive again at this time.

Weaning

As time goes by the mare increasingly restricts nursing and becomes more aggressive in her control of the foal. Nursing bouts become shorter and are usually terminated by the foal before its mother shows any aggression. The foal is increasingly responsible for any separation between the two and the mother becomes increasingly responsible for bringing them back together (Tyler, 1972). This trend continues until the time of weaning. If the mare is pregnant weaning will normally be completed shortly before the next birth, when the foal is about 40 weeks old, otherwise it may continue to suckle for a year or more (Duncan, 1980).

Normal sexual behaviour of the stallion

Stallion sexual behaviour can be considered in two broad categories:

(1) Behaviour which keeps his harem together
(2) Courtship and mating behaviour.

These will be considered in turn. The initial expression of these behaviours is largely dependent on the effects of the male hormone, testosterone, which is released from the testicles and affects the

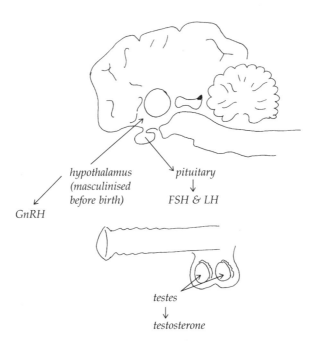

Fig. 8.4 Schematic diagram of the main endocrine organs involved in the sexual behaviour of the stallion.

brain. Such behaviours are not therefore as strong in a gelding. Some masculinisation does however occur before the foal is born, since a surge of male hormone is responsible for the development of the male genitalia; this also has a permanent effect on the brain.

Behaviour to build and maintain a harem

Within a harem the oldest mare tends to travel at the head of the group and the stallion at the rear. As explained in Chapter 7 on group behaviour, this is easier to understand if you consider the roles of different individuals in the group. By driving the mares from behind, the stallion can ensure that no mares stray and that they are less vulnerable to being kidnapped by other stallions. The stallion drives the group by running alongside but slightly behind an individual or snaking at her to move her on.

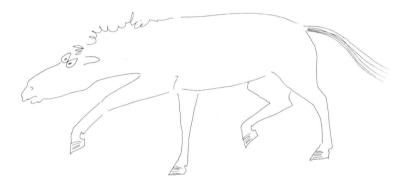

Fig. 8.5 Stallion drives mares whilst snaking his neck.

The snaking posture involves a stallion lowering and extending his head whilst laying back his ears. The head is swung from side to side or rotated like a threatening cobra.

Stray mares may be gathered into the group and other stallions driven away using this behaviour. Stallion conflicts may be preceded by a ritual display of arousal (see Figure 8.6) including foot stamping and threats, and only occasionally escalate to rearing boxing matches.

Aggression involves a risk of injury even if you are likely to win the fight. Accordingly natural selection has favoured individuals who adopt strategies which avoid such conflict. This involves the assessment of signals directly and indirectly associated with a stallion's fitness.

(1) **Direct signals** include visual ones like those described in Figure 8.6 and the audible roars.
(2) **Indirect signals** include the chemical ones left by a stallion

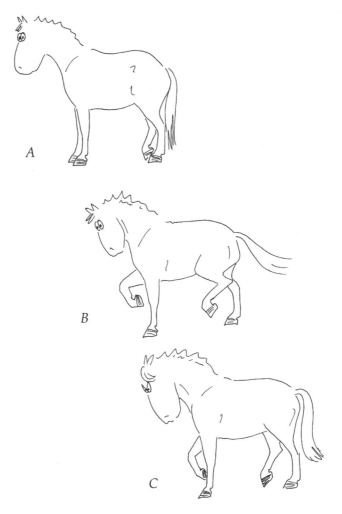

Fig. 8.6 Stallions respond to a threat with (A) increased arousal and attention to the threat, (B) a ritualised form of approach, (C) threats of physical violence.

over his territory. In this regard, as discussed in Chapter 7, the harem may be considered to be a moving territory since he will tend to mark over the urine and faeces of the other members of his harem. Faeces are particularly useful as a means of communication in your absence. We are only just beginning to appreciate the complexity of the chemical signals used, but a decent pile of faeces not only declares who you are, but also how recently you have been there. For this reason a stallion tends to defecate over his own faeces as this notifies others of his continued presence and avoids unnecessary conflict. If the

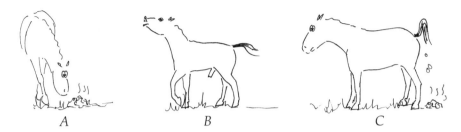

Fig. 8.7 Stallions will often flehmen in response to the eliminations of a mare and then mark over these with his own dung.

herd is non-migratory then piles of faeces will accumulate in specific sites. These are often referred to as stud piles and are commonly seen in domestic studs.

Courtship and mating behaviour

When a stallion detects that one of his mares is about to come into oestrus he may become a real nuisance, though others may be less of a problem to manage. He may drive, snake and bite the haunches of such a mare for several days if necessary. However, only if she stands still in response to this will he attempt the next stage of courtship. If the mare is receptive he will nudge and nip along her body towards her neck. Both animals may appear to behave quite aggressively to each other at this time, but this should soon settle if the mare is in oestrus. The stallion will sniff her perineum, flehmen in response to any secretion or excretion and call out with a long low nicker sound. The stallion also uses a ritual prancing gait in his courtship display (Figure 7.1). The origin of such signals has already been discussed in Chapter 7. Jerky movements increase the attention value of the display. Horses naturally attend to such movements since they have such enormous survival value at other times, for example when a predator finally decides to make a decisive strike.

If the mare responds favourably with clitoral winks, the stallion's penis is extended and will become erect. He will make several partial mounts before attempting a full mount, usually from behind but occasionally from the side. Intromission is normally achieved after a few exploratory thrusts. Copulation does not take long and, after a few pelvic thrusts, flagging of the raised tail signals ejaculation. The stallion's head also tends to lower and the facial muscles relax at this time. During copulation the stallion may bite occasionally at the mare's neck and mane. Within about 30 seconds the mare will normally step forward to allow the stallion to dismount. It is not uncommon for a stallion to squeal a little at this time. In the natural state the stallion does not have to step backwards to dismount. The stallion may be willing to serve another mare within ten minutes or so, and is likely to show mated mares greater attention over the next few days. A mare in oestrus tends to be served on five to ten occasions.

Effects of captivity

It is often considered unsafe to keep stallions together but in the wild bachelor bands are a normal feature. Why is this? Stallions will fight and possibly even kill each other when they are competing over possession of a group of females. Deaths are however not the norm and even ultimately fatal injuries are not common in the wild. A serious fight involves great risks for both parties and, as with other aggressive behaviour, an escalating series of threats is issued and physical contact only made when absolutely necessary. This may be because the two stallions are unable clearly to determine who is likely to win a contest or because the loser is unable to retreat. These situations are more likely in the domestic environment.

Stallions being kept for breeding purposes are often near mares and so there is the potential for competition when a female comes into oestrus. Stallions living together in the wild have often grown up together or shared some adolescent life. During this time they can learn about each other's strengths and weaknesses and so more fully evaluate and recognise their chances in any serious competition. In addition they learn the rules of living in a social group (see Chapter 7). Such opportunities or information are rarely available to domestic stallions and the captive environment may not allow some of the signals normally used in such evaluation to be transmitted efficiently. For example, the audible roar may be muffled or blocked by enclosed housing. Moreover, should a fight take place, a paddock may not be large enough or provide sufficient cover for the loser to retire safely. The aggression of stallions in captivity is therefore behaviour that can be expected for such an abnormal situation. The problem lies more with the management system than the horse.

Modifiers of the genetic blueprint

In this section we consider how the normal natural behaviour patterns may be altered.

Breakdowns in the chemical chain

The sexual behaviour characteristics described above are regulated by a complex internal chemistry. Both nature and man can alter this, breaking the link between the genetic programme and the hormone triggers of sexual behaviour.

Mares with disrupted cycles

It is not uncommon, especially in the latter half of the season, for a corpus luteum to fail to degenerate in the normal way. The persistence of this structure causes a prolonged dioestrus (possibly lasting several months) when the mare ceases to cycle in the normal way. Veterinary attention will normally sort out the problem sooner than this and may include the use of drugs to break down this structure.

Tumours of the ovary occasionally occur and usually disturb the normal cycle of reproductive behaviour. Oestrus cycles are usually irregular in the beginning and then stop completely. Some time after this, the mare may start to show stallion like behaviour. These effects are probably due to the effect of the hormones on pituitary control mechanisms.

Castration

The most obvious artificial intervention by man on the sexual blueprint of many horses is the castration of colts. Geldings are male insofar as they have male genitalia and some of their brain has been masculinised, but in the absence of the hormone trigger, testosterone, their latent stallion behaviour tends not to be expressed.

By far the most common reason for stallion-like behaviour in an apparent gelding is the failure of one or both testicles to descend in the normal way. Retained abdominal testes do not normally develop at the usual rate and so the onset of stallion-like behaviour may be delayed beyond normal maturity or only become apparent when the testes become cancerous.

It used to be thought that a small piece of testosterone secreting tissue was occasionally left behind at castration which led to later problems, but this appears to be a myth used to explain the behaviour of animals who in reality still have at least one testicle.

The supply of testosterone is not, therefore, the whole story underlying stallion-like behaviour in geldings. If a horse is castrated late in life or after it has some sexual experience it may retain some behaviours through learning. In all these cases, the animals can be quite dangerous and veterinary attention is essential so that a rapid diagnosis can be made before appropriate treatment started.

Hormonal effects on the embryo

In theory it is possible for the natural factors in the external environment to affect the ethological development of an animal's sexual behaviour. We have already mentioned how a surge of

androgens from the embryonic testes at a particular time of pregnancy causes an area of the developing hypothalamus in the
embryo's brain and dependent structures like the pituitary to
become male. The important trigger in this developmental period is
the general molecular structure of the hormone, not its specific
form. Oestrogens will have the same effect on the embryo, i.e. they
will cause masculinisation of the brain. This is because their
molecular structure is quite similar to that of the male sex steroid
hormone, testosterone. Females are feminine because they do not
encounter any sex hormone at this time, not because the brain is
specifically feminised.

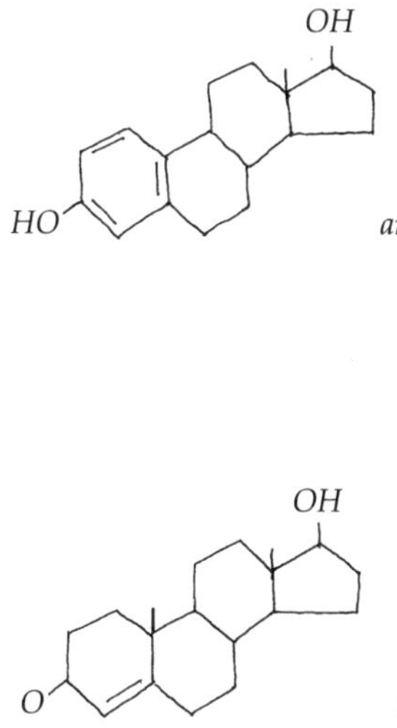

an oestrogen, oestradiol –17B

testosterone

Fig. 8.8 Molecular structure of (A) an oestrogen (B) testosterone (note
similarity).

Compounds similar to oestrogen are found in a number of
foodstuffs like lucerne and red clover, which are commonly fed to
horses. Whilst it has not been shown that their consumption during
pregnancy has any effect on the behaviour or development of female
foals, it is theoretically possible that male-like behaviour in some
fillies may have its origin in their mothers' diets during pregnancy.

The influence of previous experience

The effect of isolation
The rearing conditions of a breeding animal may have a serious
affect on its reproductive success. Stallions reared in isolation from
females can be expected to have a normal sex-drive or libido but
will often have problems with regards to orientation. They may try

to mount other males or be unsuccessful at penetrating a female. Rarely, problems may also arise as a result of abnormal primary socialisation and the horse may exhibit sexual behaviour towards another species (see the discussion on Lorenz's geese in Chapter 4).

Aversive sexual experiences

Aversive sexual experiences are not uncommon amongst both stallions and mares. This may range from supposed encouragement for the stallion actively to lift himself backwards to the use of severe punishments to stop spontaneous masturbation by the male. For mares Kiley-Worthington (1987) makes a not unreasonable comparison between the service of the hobbled and hooded mare in hand and rape.

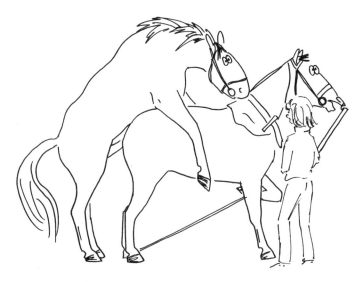

Fig. 8.9 The use of considerable restraint to service a mare 'in hand'.

Mares not in full oestrus are likely to be more overtly aggressive at this time, not through fear but through the inability to use the more gentle or subtle signals and space to move away provided by nature. Is it surprising that the mare may resist mating in future following this sort of handling or that conception rates are low? Rather than seeing this as confirmation of the need for such precautions to protect the stallion, we should maybe examine the procedure itself and look for alternatives.

Artificial management of the breeding cycle

Previous experience may also be artificially manipulated to alter the sexual behaviour patterns of horses. Whilst temperature may play a small part in determining when mares come into oestrus, day length, as described earlier, is the most important factor. Since all Thoroughbreds have their official birthday on 1 January of the year they are born and race according to age, there is some pressure to ensure that a foal is born as early in the year as possible. This is at odds with the natural cycle of day length but may be managed through the use of artificial lighting to extend the 'day' early in the season. Alternatively hormone therapy may be used to 'kick start' the system and break the link between the genetic blue-print and the normal hormonal sequence of events.

The importance of individual differences

Individuals can be differentiated on the basis of virtually any characteristic but, in a scientific context, the term 'individual differences' is used to describe stable differences in behaviour which allow individuals to be distinguished from each other but which are consistent for that individual from one time to another. With regards to sexual behaviour, one area which has been investigated is mate preference. Pickeral *et al.* (1993) have demonstrated preferences amongst mares for particular stallions. This may have some practical application for forced 'in hand' matings. It can be argued that it is adaptive for an individual to mate with others who are similar but not too similar to oneself. Individuals which are very different may not be compatible or from different geographic regions and so not as fit for the environment as more similar local individuals. On the other hand individuals who are very similar are more likely to be closely related and, as inbreeding increases the risk of genetic weaknesses being expressed, tendencies to indulge in this practice will be selected against over the generations.

Individual differences in the horse are an important area of concern which have only recently received much serious scientific attention. Horses, like people, have personality dimensions to their individuality, but we are only just beginning to understand how properly to describe and measure these traits (Mills, 1998). A timid mare may be aggressive to a stallion when in oestrus and this must be distinguished from the dioestrous mare. When we have effective methods of rating personality it may be easier for us to distinguish these situations and offer suitable sympathetic management. Perhaps the most important and exciting differences are those traits which have a clear genetic basis since these can then be selected for or bred out in order to improve the compatibility of domestic horses to their environment.

All of the above relate to part events in the individual's history or personality which affect its present behaviour. There are, of course, also many factors relating to the immediate environment which will affect the behaviour of an individual now or in the future.

The current external environment

Obviously the current environment has an essential role in shaping ongoing activity. As already discussed, mares do not show receptive behaviour in the absence of a stallion. Certain behaviours do not occur in the absence of certain stimuli, regardless of the individual's physiological state. However, the overall perception of the environment is also important in shaping the expression of behaviour. It may encourage or discourage one behaviour over others.

The effects of stress on reproduction

Stressful environments are obviously not good for optimal sexual performance. They cause the release of natural pain-killers which appear to help the individual cope with the situation. These chemicals, called enkephalins and endorphins, inhibit the release of the gonadotrophin releasing factor, which controls the release of the gonadotrophins (luteinising hormone and follicle stimulating hormone) in the pituitary. These hormones occur in both males and females and have equivalent effects in the two sexes. They directly affect the gonads, which are responsible for development and maturation of the egg and sperm. As a result of stress, there is also a fall in the levels of sex hormone (oestrogen in the mare or testosterone in the stallion) produced by the gonads. This has a direct effect on libido.

It is interesting to note that this process can also be set in motion by large amounts of regular exercise and so this should be considered when faced with a breeding problem in a working animal. However, no exercise may result in its own problems. The important thing is to get the balance right, i.e. to work with the system in the way it was designed.

Stress also results in larger amounts of prolactin being produced. This hormone is most well known for its role in milk production in the mare but it is found in both males and females and reduces the sensitivity of the pituitary to the releasing factors described above. Another group of stress hormones, the glucocorticoids, helps us prepare for the action that is normally required in order to cope with the stress. However these chemicals also reduce the sensitivity of the gonads to luteinising hormone. Therefore as a result of stress we not only have less of the sexually stimulating hormones but also a lowered sensitivity to them at a number of points along the line of action. Not only is there less interest in sex but also, over time, abnormalities such as deformed sperm in the male or irregular cycling in the female may occur.

The levels of these chemicals can be used to give an idea of the stress faced by an individual but obviously some are clearer measures than others. We will return to this theme when we talk about measuring the welfare of the horse in Chapter 10.

Stress has other detrimental effects on reproductive performance as well. When stressed the body prepares itself for action. The heart beats faster, blood pressure rises and more blood is diverted to the muscles with each beat. This process is brought about by the sympathetic nervous system (see Chapter 5). Unfortunately from the point of view of reproduction it is the opposing system, the parasympathetic nervous system, which is important in allowing the male to obtain an erect penis. The sympathetic system kicks in to allow ejaculation. For stallions therefore, stress may result in premature ejaculation at best and complete impotency at worst. An equivalent scenario can be extended to the mares which, under stress, are less keen on seeking out stallions or accepting any one that seeks them out.

Other environmental effects on reproduction

Less obvious perhaps are specific endocrinological effects from the environment. Not only can general environmental stress suppress reproduction, but the composition of a stable social environment may have a similar effect. Bachelor stallions which live in all male groups and whose only opportunity to reproduce is to be fairly sneaky about it appear to be in a different internal reproductive state to those which live with a harem. McDonnell (1996) reports that stallions kept in barns appear to have suppressed reproductive function and this may offer some of the explanation and answer for treatment.

Current health and fitness of the individual

Poor health and fitness may cause stress in the way described above but may also have more specific effects. For example, the starved mare will not only be reproductively suppressed because of the stress of her situation, but the lack of fat cells means that the small amount of testosterone which is normally produced in females can not be removed. This alone will have anti-oestrogenic effects. Factors like the level of nutrition for the animal and recovery from recent illness play an essential role in allowing an animal achieve its reproductive potential. A diet based on hay and oats may be deficient in certain amino acids which, when provided as a supplement, reduce problems associated with the sexual cycle in the mare (Bengtsson & Knudsen, 1963). Cereals do not provide a good balance of calcium and phosphorus and this too can lead to ovarian problems.

Conclusion

In this chapter we have not only described the typical sexual behaviour patterns of horses but also illustrated the sources of variation which make any specific act unique. This plan could be applied to just about any other behaviour as well. Such an approach helps us to understand and analyse the many questions we ask ourselves about why an animal is behaving in a certain way. Our only limit is the extent of our knowledge.

TOPICS FOR DISCUSSION

◇ Discuss the internal and external causal factors associated with the motivation of sexual behaviour in the mare and stallion.
◇ Compare the method of oestrus detection in the mare used by man to that of the stallion.
◇ Discuss the adaptive value of the processes of attraction and proceptivity. Are they likely to be of importance to the horse in captivity?
◇ Discuss the ethology of the bond between a mare and her new-born foal.
◇ How does the natural process of weaning compare to the managed procedures used in captivity? Discuss the possible origins of problems which might arise as a result of these differences?
◇ Consider the sources of individual variation in other equine behaviour patterns.

References and further reading

Asa, C. S. (1986) Sexual behavior of mares. In: Veterinary clinics of North America [Equine Practice] (eds Houpt, K.A. & Crowell-Davis, S.L.). *Behavior* **2** (3), 519–34.

Bengtsson, G. & Knudsen, O. (1963) Feed and ovarian activity of trotting mares in training. *Cornell Veterinarian* **53**, 404–9.

Doarn, R.T., Threlfall, W.R. & Kline, R.C. (1987) Umbilical blood flow and the effects of premature severance in the neonatal horse. *Theriogenology* **28**, 789–800.

Duncan, P. (1980) Time budgets of Camargue horses II. Time budgets of adult horses and weaned sub-adults. *Behaviour* **72**, 26–49.

Fraser, A.F. (1992) *The Behaviour of the Horse*. CAB International, Wallingford.

Ginther, O.J. (1979) *Reproductive Biology of the Mare*. McNaughton and Gun, Ann Arbor.

Hintz, H.F. (1977) Nutrition of the horse. In: *The Horse* (eds Evans, J.W., Borton, A., Hintz, H.F. & van Vleck, L.D.). Freeman, San Francisco.

Kiley-Worthington, M.(1987) *The Behaviour of Horses*. J.A. Allen, London.

McDonnell, S.M. (1996) Important lessons from free-living equids. In: *Equine Clinical Behavior*. SVPM/ASME International Congress, Basel.

Mills, D.S. (1998) Personality and individual differences in the horse, their significance, use and measurement. *Equine Veterinary Journal : Behaviour Supplement* (in Press).

Morel, M.D. (1993) *Equine Reproduction, Physiology and Stud Management*. Farming Press, Ipswich.

Pickerel, T.M., Crowell-Davis, S.L., Caudle, A.B. & Estep, D.Q. (1993) Sexual preferences of mares (*Equus caballus*) for individual stallions. *Applied Animal Behaviour Science* **38**, 1–13.

Rossdale, P.D. (1981) *Horse Breeding*. David & Charles, Newton Abbott.

Satoh, S. & Hoshi, S. (1933) A study of reproduction in the mare. Part II. The study on the oestrus. *Journal of the Japanese Society for Veterinary Science*. **12**, 200–23.

Stabenfeldt, G.H. & Edqvist, L-E. (1984) Female reproductive processes, male reproductive processes, In: Swenson M.J., (ed.) *Duke's Physiology of Domestic Animals*. 10th edn. 798–846, Cornell University Press, Ithaca.

Tyler, S. J. (1972) The behaviour and social organisation of the New Forest ponies. *Animal Behaviour Monographs* **5**, (2).

Waring, G.H. (1983) *Horse Behavior: The Behavioural Traits and Adaptations of Domestic and Wild Horses, including Ponies*. Noyes, Park Ridge.

Part 3
The Flexibility of Behaviour and its Management

So far we have considered the processes underlying the nature of the horse, i.e. what makes a horse behave like a horse. In the last part we started to explore the factors which create variations on this theme and in this part we examine the flexibility of behaviour further. We are particularly concerned with the adaptability of these traits in different environments, i.e. what a horse is capable of in even the unnatural environment of captivity. This consists of two important elements:

◇ The environment we create when we wish to train him. This includes how he responds to the different techniques used for teaching.
◇ Welfare issues connected with the normal stable environment and how he copes with the domestic existence.

We will consider each of these in turn.

9. *Learning and Training*

Psychological processes

We will start with a little history to put things in perspective.

Learning may be defined as a change in the potential to perform a behaviour as a result of experience. If there is a change in behaviour then it may be fairly easy to tell that learning has occurred, for example your horse now responds to your riding aids to trot when previously he required the assistance of learned verbal commands. However, just because he does not respond does not mean that he does not know what he should be doing. Learning is about gaining knowledge not just changing behaviour. Distinguishing between what an animal does and what it knows (i.e. what is inside its head) is a familiar problem in animal behaviour as we have seen. If we apply our own thoughts to explain what is going on then we may be accused of being anthropomorphic and unscientific.

Behaviourism

How best to study the mind was a big problem for the early psychologists. Some, such as Titchener (1896), suggested the only mind we could know was our own and therefore to understand how it worked we must concentrate on analysing our own thought processes – a procedure known as introspection. Others, like Watson (1913), criticised this process as unscientific since it could never be independently verified. He suggested that the only objective evidence we had for the minds of others was their behaviour and we should therefore concentrate on measuring behaviour in controlled situations. He was keen to see psychology develop into a respectable science and this approach led to the development of what has come to be known as the behaviourist school of psychology. This suggested a direct link between events (stimuli) and their resulting behaviour (responses). Thus a rat that learned to run a maze did so by turning a certain corner to find a reward. The behaviour of turning in that particular way was then stamped in as behavioural instructions. Eventually the rat which learns to run the maze as six steps forward followed by a right turn then ten more steps before a right turn, etc. would come to a reward. It is not suggested in this example that the rat is seeking the reward at the start, simply that the behaviour has been pre-programmed by previous experience. Continuing to reward the behaviour keeps the programme in place but does not necessarily create an expectation of reward at the start of a test, as expectation is an internal process which we cannot measure objectively.

Cognitive psychology

Unfortunately this focus on behaviour has meant that other important psychological processes such as the emotions (affect), behavioural tendencies (conation) and mental constructs (cognition) got pushed to the sidelines until more recently. However the experimental basis of cognitive psychology (as it has come to be known) goes back nearly as far as behaviourism in the writings of scientists such as Edward Tolman (1932). He showed that if you took a rat that had learned to run a maze for a reward and then flooded the maze, the rat could navigate itself to swim to the reward. Behaviour alone could not therefore be stamped in by the response, otherwise the swimming rat's behaviour should be the same as one which had no experience of the maze. This might seem fairly obvious but it highlights an important point, i.e. that there is often more than one way of explaining the acquisition of a new behaviour and this does not require consciousness or emotion.

Lloyd Morgan's Canon

Morgan (1894) suggested, in what has become known as Lloyd Morgan's Canon, that we should never seek to explain behaviour in terms of more complicated psychological processes if a simpler explanation will do. This makes a lot of sense from an evolutionary point of view. We would predict animals to exhibit the most efficient way available of achieving a goal as the less efficient ones would be selected against. It is useful when trying to determine which explanation is preferable for a given behaviour or natural occurrence, otherwise we might end up suggesting that leaves choose to jump off trees in autumn rather than simply fall as a result of biological changes in their attachment.

There is greater debate, however, over the position of higher psychological processes like consciousness and reasoning in the control of the behaviour of non-human animals. Often it is theoretically possible to explain even complex horse behaviour in terms of a long sequence of stimulus-response habits which require no thought. However we might explain such a behaviour equally well by referring to the thoughts of the horse and how its behaviour was governed by his ideas about the consequences of his actions. This may provide a shorter explanation but is it simpler? We still do not know exactly where consciousness comes from nor how certain types of thinking are achieved. We therefore often have no scientific way of supporting our suggestion that horses are thinking in a particular way.

One may ask why this matters and whether it isn't obvious that horses think. But if they do think then they think like horses not men dressed up as horses and that is much harder to imagine. This is why we need to be as objective as we can about assessing a horse's behaviour. Only then may we start to get an idea of the world from the horse's viewpoint and be able to do what is in its interest, rather than what we think is best from our own perspective. We will see later in Chapter 10 on welfare how well-meaning owners do not always provide what is best for their horse because they are giving it the same priorities as themselves. We must not be anthropomorphic in our views.

The flexible approach

The second reason why this bit of history is important relates to understanding scientific literature. Because we have two approaches to the same problem, we have two ways of explaining what is going on. Two scientists may therefore use very different terms to describe the same phenomenon. This can be a bit confusing. If you know whether or not the author is coming from a cognitive or behaviourist standpoint then you should not be surprised by the terminology used and that which is not used. Most scientists now recognise that both disciplines have something to offer and that they are not as mutually exclusive as people may have thought. The two in fact complement one another as we will see. Behaviourist style explanations help us analyse more methodically what links are being made, whilst cognitive elements help explain how this may be internally represented so that the animal has the benefit of flexibility in its learning.

A few basic procedures

Traditional texts will refer to the processes of classical (Pavlovian) and operant (Skinnerian) conditioning as the basis of learning. These are, however, only two illustrations of learning apparent from changes in behaviour and do not cover all the phenomena as we will see.

Classical conditioning

This is getting an established behaviour to occur in response to a new range of stimuli.

The process is also known as Pavlovian or respondent conditioning. The term Pavlovian comes from the Russian physiologist, Ivan Pavlov, who demonstrated the process in his laboratory dogs. Pavlov was interested in the study of saliva flow and was collecting samples in response to food. However, during his experiments he noticed that after a few trials the dogs would start to salivate before they were presented with any food. The sight of the technician that normally fed them was enough to get the juices flowing. The dogs had learned to associate the technician with food. In order to investigate the extent of this phenomenon further, Pavlov conducted experiments whereby he rang a buzzer each time the dogs were about to be fed. After a few trials he found that the dogs would salivate whenever they heard the bell even if no food followed.

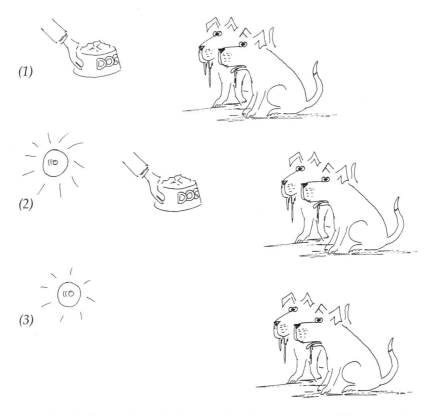

Fig. 9.1   (1) Unconditional stimulus (food) and response. (2) Association of unconditional stimulus and conditional stimulus (bell). (3) Conditional response to conditional stimulus alone.

Pavlov described the salivation in response to the presence of food as an 'unconditional response' because it was a normal, natural, biological response and did not need to be learned. The food was then an 'unconditional stimulus'. The buzzer was a 'conditional stimulus' because it did not initially elicit the salivation. However during training the presentation of food was conditional upon the buzzer sounding first. When salivation occurred in response to the buzzer without food, this activity was referred to as a 'conditional response'.

Alternative explanations
So what is happening?

(1)   We could say that the dog is learning that the buzzer predicts the food (a cognitive explanation).
(2)   Alternatively we could make a more detailed analysis and suggest that some form of association is being made. This is a behavioural or associationist explanation. The link may be between:
  ◇ the two stimuli – which suggests that the buzzer stimulus comes to be processed the same way as the food stimulus and the normal response will then occur (stimulus substitution theory); or
  ◇ the conditional stimulus and the response – which would imply that the delivery of food rewards reinforces the salivation which occurs after the sound of the buzzer (response substitution theory).

Implications for training and management
These behavioural explanations involve significant theoretical distinctions with different practical implications for considering the most effective way to train a horse. It is therefore important that we work out what is really happening. Response substitution theory suggests that the reward is important in establishing the response rather than the relationship between the two stimuli. The evidence across species tends to suggest that this is not the case and that stimulus substitution is the more common mechanism for this type of learning.

A response is transferred most effectively to a new stimulus when that stimulus is very reliably paired with the old controlling stimulus. It is preferable for the conditional stimulus to precede the unconditional stimulus (buzzer then food) and for the two to be closely related in time and space, i.e. 'contiguous'. Reverse or 'backward conditioning' (food then buzzer) is possible but takes longer to establish. This may reflect the fact that the conditional stimulus is no longer predictive of the unconditional stimulus. The unconditional response is likely to have already begun by the time the conditional stimulus appears and so the association is likely to be of less adaptive value to the animal.

The range of responses which can be classically conditioned to new stimuli include the emotional ones, as any veterinary surgeon can testify. Animals tend to avoid pain (unconditional stimulus) and impending pain generates a fear response (unconditional response). So what happens if the only time your horse sees the vet he does something painful or uncomfortable to it? The horse may be classically conditioned to be fearful of the vet. There are specific techniques used in the treatments of fears and phobias as we will see below but if the fear is not too intense this problem can be quite simply treated and prevented. Ask the vet to give a treat to all the horses on the yard whether or not he has had to treat them. This way he is no longer predictive of something nasty. A non-frightened horse is easier, quicker and safer to treat.

From an adaptive point of view classical conditioning allows an animal to anticipate events and so be prepared for changes in the environment.

Operant conditioning

This describes the process of learning to do something differently.

A bit more history – the law of effect

Thorndike (1898) discovered that, if he put hungry cats in a box where they had to press a lever to escape and get some food, the time taken for them to escape shortened with experience. Eventually they learned to perform the behaviour which led to their escape as soon as they were placed in the box. Initially their behaviour was random and they would 'accidentally' hit the release lever, but with time it became more focused.

Thorndike referred to this as 'trial error and accidental success' learning and it led him to propose the law of effect. This states that: a response that is followed by a reward is more likely to recur whereas one that is followed by an unpleasant experience is less likely to occur again.

This type of learning has many other names such as instrumental learning, since the behaviour is 'instrumental' in affecting the response that follows. The term operant conditioning comes from the psychologist B. F. Skinner who studied the effects of reward and punishment on operant behaviours. He defined these as behaviours that were not particularly tied to any stimulus (unlike salivation, which is tied to the presence of things like food and so is called a 'respondent' behaviour). His extensive work in this field has led some people to refer to the process as 'Skinnerian learning'.

What makes a reward and or punishment?

Operant conditioning allows the modification of behaviour as a result of its consequences and so has enormous adaptive advantages to the animal. It not only occurs in training when we deliberately use rewards and punishments but whenever an animal does something of any consequence. It is how the environment feeds back onto behaviour. The underlying principle is that of 'reinforcement'. Reinforcement may be defined as: those events following a behaviour which affect its future performance in similar circumstances.

There is a lot of confusion and inconsistency in the use of several important terms used to describe reinforcement and its effects. So we will define them as we introduce them. Reinforcers may be divided into two groups:

(1) **Appetitive reinforcers** which increase the likelihood of a behaviour with which they are associated, i.e. they are forms of reward
(2) **Aversive reinforcers** which have the opposite effect reducing the likelihood of a behaviour with which they are associated, i.e. punishment.

Beware that some texts use the term 'reinforcer' to describe only appetitive reinforcers. The effect of a reinforcer depends on how it is perceived by the horse not its intended effect by a handler.

Failure to appreciate this can lead to a number of problems, as we shall see. If we go to collect a horse from a field with other horses, call it and immediately lead it away to a solitary box, what have we taught the horse? Come to me when I call and I will isolate you from your companions. This is not a great reward for obedience. Should we be surprised therefore when the horse becomes difficult to catch up from the field? The way round this problem is to always give your horse a reward when it comes. This need not be a food treat, indeed, in this case it may be preferable to give the horse a good rub on the withers as this is a recognisable social greeting which seems to be inherently rewarding for the horse. Also sometimes call your horse up just for a rub and a chat in this way, not only when you want to take him away to the stable.

The reinforcement process

Appetitive reinforcers to encourage a specific behaviour may work through either positive or negative reinforcement.

Note, these are both processes which encourage a certain

behaviour. The difference between these two types of reinforcement is a relative one. Some psychologists argue that they represent fundamentally the same process. If an ordinarily desired reward is provided in association with a behaviour then positive reinforcement is being applied. In negative reinforcement, an unpleasant (aversive) stimulus or punisher is applied until the animal performs the desired behaviour. The reward in this instance is the removal of the unpleasant stimulus – in people this is associated with a sense of relief.

Although a punisher is used in this process, it is not punishment as it is focused on increasing the occurrence of a specific behaviour, usually the escape or avoidance behaviour. As a result of negative reinforcement an animal learns to escape from an unpleasant experience by performing a specific behaviour (escape conditioning). With time the animal may learn to avoid the unpleasant situation altogether as it adopts the appropriate behaviour at the first sign of the punisher. This is called 'avoidance conditioning'. This can be made more effective by pairing the punisher with a suitable non-threatening signal in order to bring about classical conditioning to the signal. The horse then learns to show the appropriate avoidance behaviour on command.

Negative reinforcement is very commonly used with horses. Response to the bit and spur are learned in this way. For example in order to turn left bit pressure is applied with the left rein. The horse will naturally turn its head towards the left in order to try and reduce the pressure (escape behaviour). If the horse is being schooled properly the bit pressure is only released when the horse turns its head and body to the left (escape conditioning). When this rule is applied consistently the horse learns to turn left with only a slight increase in feel down the left rein (avoidance conditioning).

We have rewarded the horse's natural avoidance mechanisms in order to be able to use them to control him. If the horse is poorly schooled or given over to novices who fail to release the pressure accurately and consistently then the horse may become dull mouthed. The use of the bit inconsistently is more like a punishment; i.e. it reduces the ongoing behaviour without constructively directing an alternative behaviour towards a specific goal.

The practical and effective difference between punishment and negative reinforcement relates to the timing of the aversive stimulus in relation to the behaviour affected. As with classical conditioning the contiguity of reinforcement is critical in determining the effect of any reinforcers. In most circumstances, rewards should be provided within about half a second of the goal being achieved. The closer the association the easier it is to make. Consistency is the key.

Biological preparedness

In much the same way that it is easier for a horse to make an association between a behaviour and reinforcement closely linked in time to it, animals also tend to find it easier to make certain associations. This phenomenon has been called biological preparedness (Seligman, 1970) and suggests that animals may be neurologically wired up to make certain associations more easily. This has the advantage of making it easier for an animal to learn relevant information and less likely that it will learn irrelevant information. The biological advantage of such a system within the natural environment is obviously enormous. Efficient learners survive; slow learners get eaten.

This can be used in training. If we ask a horse to come to us we are evoking a social response, perhaps the best way to reinforce this is to use a social reward. This might take the form of a bit of mutual grooming with the fingertips over the withers. Similarly a social punishment such as walking away and leaving your horse alone, might be used for a socially unacceptable behaviour like an overenthusiastic reciprocation of the mutual grooming. However, we must be careful in this situation to distinguish between a horse biting because it is clumsy with its mouth and one which is biting to stop us from doing something. In the latter case leaving the horse, rewards the misbehaviour and makes it more likely to occur in similar situations.

Punishment perceived as a reward

The object of punishment is to stop or reduce the likelihood of an ongoing behaviour. Many handlers readily use it but often inappropriately. It is worth re-emphasising that rewards and punishers are defined by their effect not by their intended action. Not uncommonly handlers may end up rewarding a behaviour that they are intending to punish. Consider the horse that kicks the door for attention. Many yard managers end up shouting at the horse for engaging in this annoying habit. The horse stops and they may think that their verbal reprimand has been an effective punishment. This situation could however be viewed differently. If this horse were kicking the door for attention, then we would expect the horse to stop when it achieves its goal. Attention takes many forms including a simple acknowledgement of your existence which might be a swear word thrown in your direction.

How can we tell whether or not the door banging has been rewarded or punished by the manager's action? The answer lies in the long-term changes in behaviour. Does the horse decrease its tendency to kick the door when the yard manager is about? Horses have a strong social tendency (Chapter 7) and the reality of the situation is that most of these activities seem to be attention related. We shall discuss how best to manage this problem below.

The effects of different reinforcement schedules

A reinforcement schedule describes when reinforcement should be applied to a behaviour and has important implications for its effectiveness. Skinner gained much of this information from experiments on rats and pigeons in order to propose general laws which could be applied to any species, including horses. These general laws form the basis of any sound training regime. Simple schedules are described below.

Continuous reinforcement

This means that each and every response is reinforced. If appetitive reinforcement is used the response is strengthened each time and the new behaviour established rapidly. This is normally used in the early stages of training in order to establish the new response. However if this is used alone, then the horse soon stops performing when we stop rewarding. This loss of a response is known as 'extinction'.

Extinction schedule

This is the opposite of continuous reinforcement and means that no responses are reinforced. It eventually leads to reduction of the unacceptable behaviour to an unreliable or unpredictable level. During this process the behaviour may become more variable which may mean that it becomes more intense or exotic before it disappears. Behaviours, which were previously reinforced, reappear at this time (resurgence), possibly in an attempt by the animal to re-establish some form of reward. Other behaviour changes seen at this time include signs which seem to indicate emotional frustration, including aggression. Accordingly a reinforced behaviour problem may appear to become worse initially if an attempt is made to eliminate it by extinction alone. Once a behaviour has been successfully reduced by extinction, the effect is not necessarily permanent. The behaviour may be subject to 'spontaneous recovery' if a long interval passes between the session when extinction was achieved and the next opportunity for the behaviour.

We will return to our door banging horse for an illustration of this point. We could choose to ignore the behaviour in the hope that it stops. If we do this we must be prepared for it to worsen before it improves and ensure that we stay on the yard until it stops. We should not be surprised if it recurs next time we are on the yard but it should be extinguished more quickly the next time. Eventually

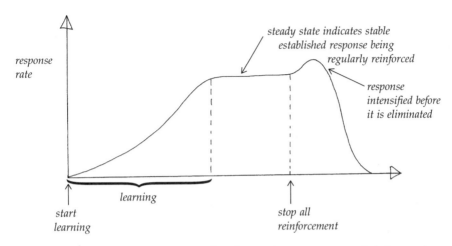

Fig. 9.2 Graph illustrating the change in a response as it is learned through reinforcement and then extinguished by non-reinforcement.

through repeated extinction schedules the behaviour will be eliminated.

Intermittent schedules
These lie between these extremes. They may be fixed or, more commonly, variable. In a fixed schedule the response to be rein-forced is specified but in a variable schedule it is only specified that a certain response should be reinforced a certain number of times on average. A fixed ratio schedule of five would suggest that every fifth response is reinforced, whereas as variable ratio of five means that the third, seventh, eleventh and twentieth responses may be reinforced (the twentieth response brings the fourth reinforcement, i.e. an average of five responses per reinforcement). This more flexible approach means that rewards can be applied to the better examples of the behaviour to be reinforced. Also since none of us are perfectly consistent, variable schedules are a more realistic option than fixed ones, although an effort should be made to maintain the planned rate of reward.

Skinner showed that intermittent schedules are better in several ways than continuous ones and these make them particularly useful when trying to train any animal to perform a particular task.

(1) **Longer sessions** More training is possible in a single session because less reinforcement is used for each correct response. For example, if carrots are used as a reward for a horse, there will come a time when the horse no longer sees carrots as something desir-able. At this point it is said that the horse has become satiated with the intended reinforcer and it ceases to be reinforcing. If the limit

were five carrots and one carrot given for each correct response, five responses could be reinforced on a continuous schedule, but twenty responses could be reinforced with an intermittent schedule of four.

(2)   **More persistent results** Intermittently reinforced behaviours are more persistent and more resistant to extinction (see above). This means that when something has been learned as a result of intermittent reinforcement, the response seems to be remembered better and is more vigorous.

(3)   **More focused training** Intermittent reinforcement on a variable schedule can be used to shape behaviour towards a specific goal. This means that, if we are trying to train a horse to do something quite difficult, by only rewarding the better examples the performance improves more rapidly (see below).

It takes an animal longer to learn a given task using intermittent schedules but this problem can be overcome by initially using a continuous schedule to demonstrate what is required and then rapidly moving over to an intermittent schedule. This will ensure rapid acquisition and effective retention of newly learned tasks.

Other simple intermittent schedules include interval and duration (time) schedules.

(1)   **A duration schedule** demands that the behaviour be performed continuously for a stated time period before it is reinforced. It teaches the animal to keep trying despite the effort required.

(2)   **An interval schedule** is where the response is only reinforced when it occurs at least a certain time after the last reinforced response. A fixed interval of five minutes means that the first response that occurs at least five minutes since the time of the last reinforcement is reinforced. Similarly, variable intervals are possible in the laboratory setting. These tend not be used so much in practice. However if you only have a few pieces of carrot, which you want to use in your training, you can divide the session into a number of intervals with only one reward available in each.

Applying reinforcement to train new behaviours

When we want to teach a horse a new behaviour efficiently, we should aim to reinforce every occurrence of the behaviour initially and then move reinforcement onto an intermittent schedule. In this way the behaviour will be rapidly learned and remembered well. In order to do this, the horse must achieve the goal in order for it to be rewarded. This does not always happen, and an alternative strategy must be used. The two most commonly used are described below.

Successive approximation

For some behaviours, such as jumping a fence, the final behavioural goal can be worked towards in stages. In these cases reinforcement may be used to shape the behaviour towards the goal by a process known as successive approximation or shaping. Imagine that you want to teach your horse to jump fences, remember the modern horse evolved on the large grasslands where their chief defence is their size combined with their speed. It is not normal for a horse to go over an obstacle as it would normally go round it.

If the horse does not jump we cannot reinforce the behaviour directly. So what do we do? We may start by simply asking the horse to go over some trotting poles. This can be done by loose schooling him. In this way there is no rider to distract him or possibly send confusing signals. Using a verbal cue like 'over' will help tell the horse that he is being asked to do something special or different. This is a discriminatory stimulus. As the horse learns to go over, we reward him every time. Simple praise and a pat will do. We then raise the pole slightly off the ground and continue as before. You approach, tell him 'over' and reward him for succeeding. If he refuses, you can ask again, but beware as you may be asking too much too soon. In this case you will need to go back a step.

As long as he can get over from a standing start, do not let him turn away. If there are any problems, the jump can be positioned alongside a solid wall and a fence constructed parallel to this to form an alleyway. He can then be gently driven forward over the jump more easily.

As he becomes more accomplished at a small jump, switch to intermittent reinforcement before you raise the jump any higher. You now only reward those jumps which are particularly neat in their take-off and/or landing. This way he learns that he must not just jump, but that he must do so in a particular way. The intermittent use of reinforcement in this way will lead him to alter his own behaviour as his brain works out what is getting rewarded and what is not. It is far easier to sort out style at this early stage than to alter a technique which has become well established and only gives problems with the higher jumps.

When he is reliably performing well we make the jump a little harder and introduce the rider. The voice cue can then be used if he ever becomes 'spooky' or indecisive. This is most likely to happen when you introduce new forms of jump or higher jumps. It allows him to discriminate when you want him to go over and when you do not, which is why it is known as a 'discriminatory stimulus'. Without this, you might end up with a horse that simply refuses to jump certain fences because going round seems a better option to him. Just as your voice may help your horse to discriminate between the options when there may be some confusion, so might other stimuli. For this reason, it is important to make sure you vary the form and colour of jumps at each stage. Otherwise he may end up learning that 'over' means jump the nearest red and white pole. By providing variation, our horse learns that 'over' means jump whatever is in front. The response has now generalised. Response generalisation is an important component to good fluid, confident action.

As an effective trainer you must maintain your position as controller and apply the three Cs:

(1) **Communicate** – the voice command tells him what he should do
(2) **Co-ordinate** – apply the aids correctly to reinforce this command
(3) **Cohere** – if you reward him appropriately, he will want to respond to you.

As he becomes more confident and able, he will learn to discriminate more subtle signals than a voice command. He will prepare to jump when you want him to even before you think you have asked him. If required, you can start to drop out the command word by giving it ever more quietly. This process is known as 'fading'. Incidentally, this sensitivity and ability of horses to pick out the most subtle of discriminatory stimuli explains why some owners think that their horse must have some form of sixth sense. We do not need to use such a fancy explanation, we just need to appreciate how we are adapting his refined survival skills for our own aims.

Behaviour chaining

Some tasks are more complicated and may be learned more efficiently by using a technique known as behaviour chaining. It is most often used to teach complex behaviour sequences, for example in performing animals in the circus or in films. In these circumstances you do not want to give a series of commands but want the horse to do a number of actions one after the other.

Suppose we want to teach a horse to open its door walk across the yard and switch on the light. We would have to wait a long time if we had to wait until the horse just happened to do it and then rewarded it. In this case we teach each of the components separately, with a discriminatory stimulus command and reward according to a continuous schedule. We will often concentrate on the last act first. When two sequences that must occur successively are being performed efficiently, we put them together; we give the command for the first and then the second. These two commands are then always paired and the horse will soon learn through a process of classical conditioning that one always precedes the other. Before long he will be starting the second sequence before you can instruct him. At this point you should start to drop the second command and reward him each time. As he learns to perform reliably, you can move to an intermittent reward at the end of the sequence.

There are several techniques for building up a response chain.

(1) Start at the end and slowly work sequence by sequence to the start.
(2) Start at both ends and slowly work toward the middle before joining the whole act together into one long sequence.
(3) Build several small pairs or clusters of actions and once established, start to amalgamate them cluster by cluster.

Individual horses, trainers and tasks all affect which technique is most appropriate. It is best to start with the one which you feel suits you best and try the others if you seem to be having difficulty.

If we wanted to teach the trick described above, we might try the following. Place a treat on the switch and introduce the horse to it, then give a command. As he investigates the switch he is likely to click it. This is then rewarded with plenty of praise and contact. You may need to add an extension to the switch so that he has something larger to work with initially. This can be faded out later. It will also help if you can repeat the command just before the switch is triggered if you can tell that it is about to occur.

Train him to walk from his box to the switch. This is not difficult if he already associates the area with food.

During other training sessions around the same time, shape his behaviour so he learns to slide the bolt across at the top of his door. Painting some treacle on the bolt and rewarding him with some more food when the bolt slides back can achieve this quite easily. Remember that if you use a different command for each of these actions it will be easier to control the behaviours. When each of the last two actions is being performed reliably on command they may be joined together. (He may in fact do this himself.) Once this sequence is established start in the box with the door opening command. As he opens the door give the second command. You should reintroduce a continuous schedule at the end of the sequence at this point. Soon he will perform the whole sequence on command and you can move back onto an intermittent schedule.

In this example individual commands for each step may not be strictly necessary, but they are important if you want to train more complex tricks using the same principles. Your only limit is your imagination and the safety of all involved; but remember, if you teach your horse a trick, do not be surprised if he does it other times. Teaching horses to open their stable door can lead to problems; you will always have a horse who is capable of letting himself out if you do not use some other 'horse-proof' lock on the door.

Punishment and its problems

Punishment is an integral part of the learning process but there are many problems with its use as a training aid. As a result it tends to be misused and so causes a lot of concern to people who have the horse's welfare at heart. Punishment should not be confused with the use of punishers in order to achieve negative reinforcement of a specific behaviour (see above).

Problems with punishment as a training aid are considered in more detail below.

Lack of focus

Punishment is not a particularly efficient training tool, as it does not specifically tell the horse what it should be doing. It just signals that one specific activity in a given context should not be performed. Since there are more ways to get something wrong than to get it right, one undesired behaviour may be exchanged for another if the appropriate behaviour is not specifically encouraged by appetitive reinforcement.

If we paint an area of chewed wood with a bitter treatment, the horse may well avoid the treated areas but we should not be surprised if he chews wood elsewhere. In fact we may paradoxically be encouraging wood chewing when we only paint certain areas. If the horse is used to chewing wood and we start to treat some areas with a bitter paint, what happens from a psychological perspective? Areas that used to be chewed now become aversive, but the bitter taste is not strong enough to stop all chewing. After all the horse has learned that some of the wood in its stable has tasted good for the last few months. Eventually the horse is likely to chew a new area which has not been treated. Imagine the relief of finding a nice piece of fresh wood to chew! Wood chewing is not effectively punished, but negative reinforcement for chewing wood in specific areas may be occurring. The behaviour may therefore paradoxically increase in the new areas. If punishment is to be effective it must be used on a continuous basis, i.e. all surfaces must be effectively made aversive, until the behaviour has been controlled. For the same reason, handlers should not punish behaviours which can occur in their absence. Otherwise a general problem may become an owner absent one. For example, there is no point in smacking your horse every time you see him chew wood, at best you are only likely to stop him chewing when you are there.

Aversion to the handler

Handler centred punishment may also result in avoidance of the handler by classical conditioning. If punishment is perceived to be delivered by a particular person, such as the owner, rather than as a direct consequence of the behaviour, the person will become a conditioned punisher. The handler is then avoided whenever he or she approaches the horse. Also, if the horse is concentrating on escape, due to escape conditioning, it is not in the best state of mind to learn something new from the handler. The horse may then be regarded as difficult or useless as it is restless or tries to escape from the handlers whenever they go near it.

Habituation

Repeated use of punishment reduces its effectiveness. Physical punishment causes discomfort and an increase in arousal within an individual – a 'startle' or 'sit up and take notice' response. If this or any other reflexive behaviour is repeatedly triggered, the response starts to weaken. This phenomenon is known as 'habituation' and is a simple form of learning affecting reflexive behaviours. This should not be confused with the extinction of a learned response (see above). Habituation and its consequences are important when we consider how people tend to use punishment. If a horse misbehaves, it is not unusual to be concerned that you might hurt or upset your horse if you use too much force. As a result most people tend to use only a very mild physical rebuke. If this is not an adequate punisher, the horse may show a startle response, i.e. take note of you, but continue to be a problem. If the same or only slightly more intense punishment is used, then the horse will start to habituate to the supposed punishments. As a result the owner may be caught up in a steadily increasing spiral of punishment, until it becomes unacceptably harsh. It may be thought that the horse is stubborn or stupid but he has become punishment resistant because of his treatment. The problem is that the punishment procedure was not adequate. A punisher should be effective the first time it is used. In this way a less severe punishment is required in the long run.

Aggression and learned helplessness

Punishment inhibits learning, and if used excessively emotional changes may occur which can give serious cause for concern. Perhaps the most common manifestation of this is some form of aggression. People who use punishment as a training method may then exacerbate an aggressive horse further.

An alternative emotional response to excessive or inconsistent punishment has been described behaviourally as 'learned helplessness' and may be similar to some forms of depression in people. It would seem that if any animal has no apparent way consistently to find a reward, then it learns that it has no control over its environment and appears to give up on trying to do anything. This may be particularly common in the badly ridden horse which is constantly being jabbed in the mouth. If it does not habituate to the random tugs on its mouth, then it may give up trying to respond to any amount of bit pressure. Once again the unfortunate response of some riders reflects a failure to examine their role in the problem. The horse may be labelled as stupid and/or stubborn, which again exacerbates the problem.

Increased timidity

Punishment makes a fearful horse worse. Punishment produces an aversion to doing a particular behaviour and emotionally this may be represented by feelings of fear. What happens then if we punish a scared horse? Imagine someone holding a horse whilst a vet tries to take a blood sample from it. The horse is scared and starts to become agitated. The handler punishes the horse in an attempt to stop it from 'misbehaving'. The pain caused by this punishment reinforces the horse's desire to escape because something unpleasant is going on. Next time the horse is likely to be even more scared and who knows how it will react then? Punishment should avoided in these circumstances. The horse should be calmed, if necessary away from the vet and then distracted whilst the work is done. In the longer term the fear may need treating with specific psychological techniques like systematic desensitisation (see below).

Potentially an abuse

In conclusion, punishment is a normal instructive part of learning, but it does not produce specific behaviours. It is therefore an inefficient training tool and should not be used as the basis of teaching a new behaviour. It is often difficult or impossible to apply appropriately in many situations, but easy to misuse. The misuse of punishment represents an abuse of the horse.

General guidelines to training new behaviours

(1) Seek opportunities for positive reinforcement, as these direct the animal's behaviour towards a precise training goal.
(2) Remember reinforcers are defined by their effect not their intended purpose. If a horse is satiated with a reinforcer then it is no longer a reinforcer.

(3)   Choose an appropriate schedule for the training programme.
(4)   Be selective about which behaviours are to be reinforced. This helps you to apply reinforcement appropriately.
(5)   The choice of reinforcer should be as relevant as possible in order to take advantage of the biological biases within the horse, e.g. social greetings.
(6)   Be careful of contiguity factors. If we give a horse food in response to a nudge, we may be training the horse to push us rather than come to us. Similarly if we punish an animal when it stops misbehaving (possibly because we cannot get near it while it is causing problems) we may be punishing the animal for stopping the problem behaviour.
(7)   Secondary reinforcers, including verbal praise and retort, must be classically conditioned to an appetitive or aversive reinforcer before they have any effect on the behaviour. Although the tone of voice might convey something do not expect a horse to understand English; it is your job as the trainer to try and understand Horse.

Learning beyond a change in behaviour

Learning is most apparent when there is a change in an animal's behaviour. This behaviour change may be manifested as a change in:

(1)   The form of the behaviour (topography of response)
(2)   The number of errors made
(3)   The strength of the response
(4)   The speed of the response
(5)   The delay in the response (latency to act)
(6)   The frequency with which the behaviour occurs (response rate).

Any of these may be used as measures when trying to determine whether or not learning is occurring and, if so, what is being learned. However, the development of cognitive psychology has led many people to recognise that not all learning is demonstrated by a change in behaviour, since circumstances may never require an animal to show everything it knows. How many times have you learnt things for an exam, only to find that they never came up on the paper itself, but you still remember these obscure facts even though you are unlikely ever to need to reproduce something as bizarre as Avogadro's constant!

Learning is about gaining knowledge and making new associations. In this way the analytical approach of behaviourism can be very useful in describing the range of associations which can be made. This is vital when trying to understand the effects of training or analyse the origins of a problem. It is perfectly reasonable to recognise this structure to learning whilst also accepting that there may be a variety of psychological mechanisms underlying similar associations.

Sea slugs with only a few thousand neurones have been shown to demonstrate a form of habituation to mild electric shocks. The mechanism for this is likely to be very different to that which underlies habituation by a cat to a complex noise. Nonetheless, the fact that some form of habituation can be demonstrated in such a simple animal with no consciousness, might suggest to some that consciousness is not necessary for any form of habituation. From this they may be happy to accept that non-human animals are not conscious. This is not a logical argument but neither can it be proved that any animal is conscious as we know it.

Learned associations

Listed below is a range of associations seen in learning which have previously been described by authors such as Walker (1987). Not all of these are obvious from an immediate behavioural response, but they suggest what might happen when there is some contiguity between two events. We must be aware of this so that we can analyse what we are teaching a horse and what a horse might learn from its environment.

To say a response or stimulus has 'motivational significance' implies that it has some inherent reinforcing property or natural effect on the underlying 'drive'.

Stimulus – stimulus (not motivationally significant)

This represents associations between stimuli which are of no motivational significance. This sort of learning occurs when we remember the layout of various things in a field. It is often called behaviourally silent or latent learning since although it is not immediately apparent that any learning has occurred, this knowledge may be used at a later date and so a difference is then apparent. Having run around a field a horse may then know where it is preferable to look for shelter when it is required. The horse has not in this case found the shelter whilst actively seeking or needing it but has stored the information for later use.

Stimulus – motivationally significant stimulus

This is the forming of an association between a motivationally significant stimulus, e.g. food and one which is not initially of the same significance, e.g. the time of day. This is what happens in classical conditioning. The result is that the stimulus which was not of primary motivational significance (conditional stimulus) comes to evoke the same response as the motivationally significant one (unconditional stimulus) (see Figure 9.1).

Stimulus – response (not motivationally significant)
If a stimulus reliably precedes a certain response, then the behaviour may become a habit to that stimulus. For example if we tell a horse 'foot up' and then pick the foot up, it is possible by simple repetition alone to get the horse to raise its foot when we use this command. The command and the response have become linked without any reward.

Response – motivationally significant stimulus
In this situation a previously insignificant behaviour is linked to a motivationally significant stimulus. This is what happens when we happen to find out that if we do something specific it will lead to a certain goal. This leads to the development of goal directed behaviour. For example a horse may learn where the feed bin is by trial and error and then actively seek it out. It is one of the associations seen in operant conditioning (see above).

Response – motivationally significant response
Sometimes just doing a behaviour has an effect on our motivational state. Some things we enjoy doing, others we loathe and yet others we do not care about one way or the other. Those behaviours of motivational significance, can be used to reinforce other behaviours which were previously of no significance. A reward for doing something right may then be another enjoyable behaviour or a punishment could be having to do something which is normally avoided. Premack (1959) suggested, in what has become known as 'the Premack Principle', that any desirable behaviour which occurs less frequently than another may be used as a reinforcer. After a period of intense training with a horse it may be worth allowing it to literally 'horse around' for a while by way of reward for all the hard work. These sorts of association are also seen in some forms of operant conditioning.

Response – stimulus (not motivationally significant)
Some behaviours have consequences which are not of any general motivational significance to the behaviour itself but are more informative about the consequences of the behaviour. For example, a horse may learn how to untie its hay net.

Response – response (not motivationally significant)
In the same way that a certain stimulus may become linked to a specific response to form a habit, one response may be associated

with another. This forms the basis of many performance skills. Skilful action does not allow pause for thought between the behaviours making up the behavioural sequence. If one action is always followed by another the horse may learn the routine by repetition without any reward. If you always hack out on the same route, some horses seem to need no instruction as to what to do as soon as you leave the yard.

Analysis and application

When you are training a horse, consider the type of associations which you are seeking to establish. Are they easy and clear for the horse to understand? If so, then he should learn quickly. Just as important is to stop and think what is happening when he does not respond well or seems to misbehave. Look at his behaviour and see what associations are being made. If you can recognise the associations you can ask yourself why they are being made. You are then halfway to solving the problem. Learning does not lie.

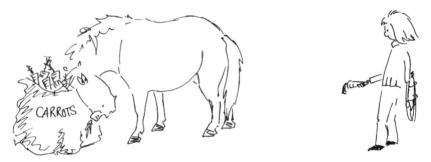

Fig. 9.3 Rewards for an alternative behaviour must provide more benefit than that provided by the ongoing behaviour.

Training techniques for problem behaviours

The study of experimental and clinical psychology has allowed us to develop reliable techniques for behavioural modification in the management of a range of behaviour problems. We will describe and illustrate a few of them here. They should be used with care and, if you are in any doubt, then you should seek expert assistance.

Flooding

This may used to treat a horse which is over-sensitive for some reason, for example one that is scared unnecessarily or one that gets over-excited easily in response to certain stimuli or events.

Flooding may be used for the treatment of fears and phobias, but this procedure is not without risk. Serious consideration should be given to the horse's welfare before it is used.

A simple example will illustrate the point. If you have an irrational fear of spiders, you could be cured by being thrown into a small room full of spiders and left there until you cope and realise that there is nothing really to fear after all. You habituate to the situation. Sometimes, however, this technique does not work, particularly if the fear is unusually severe. In these cases the treatment would represent an uncontrollably massive punishment and you might respond with a state of learned helplessness (see above) and become quite simply a blubbering wreck.

Like all forms of learning, habituation may be forgotten and so it is important to reinforce the learning on an occasional basis.

There are several important principles to flooding, which must be recognised if it is to be used effectively in the horse.

(1)   Suitable cases must be chosen with care and due consideration for the horse's well-being. Flooding should not be used if you are not fully confident that you have the facilities to complete the programme of treatment.

(2)   The horse should be exposed to the exciting stimulus in an environment where it cannot escape from it and cannot cause injury.

(3)   The horse and stimulus should be left together until the horse habituates to the stimulus. This is indicated by the return of normal behaviour and normal resting physiological parameters like heart rate and respiration rate. If this does not happen, the horse is likely to have become even more sensitised to the problem as a result of negative reinforcement.

(4)   The process should then be repeated several times in a variety of suitable locations in order to prevent loss of the habituation response. This loss is technically known as 'dishabituation'. This is most likely if too long a time gap is left between sessions or if the same treatment area is used each time. If the original response does reappear, then it should be eliminated more easily on a repeat programme of treatment.

(5)   The learning process should be reinforced frequently. It is very frustrating to cure a horse of its fear of being clipped only to find yourself back at square one the next year. The horse does not need to be clipped in the summer, only exposed to the routine, noise and feel of the clippers.

Scared horses can be very dangerous. On no account should the animal be physically punished when it is scared as this is likely to make the situation worse.

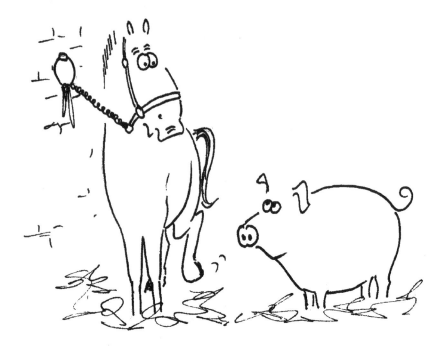

Fig. 9.4   Flooding.

An illustration of flooding for the control of a horse's fear of pigs is shown in Figure 9.4. This is not to be recommended!

Systematic desensitisation

This is a more humane way of dealing with problems similar to those which respond to flooding. Unfortunately, though, this process takes longer and is not always practical. Wolpe (1958) developed systematic desensitisation as a technique for treating phobias in people. It involves training the patient to relax, whilst some aspect, but not the whole body, of the fear-provoking stimulus is introduced. The patient is trained to relax in the presence of several different components of the problem before they are joined together one stage at a time. The patient is constantly reinforced for remaining relaxed at this time. Eventually the patient stays calm in the presence of the full problem stimulus. A development of this technique is to get the patient to tense up before they are required to relax during the training session, this seems to produce a greater relaxation. In the horse this can be achieved by exercising him first. Suppose your horse is scared of pigs, a systematic desensitisation programme might be as follows:

(1) **Lunge or free-school the horse.** Do this until you have worked up a bit a sweat on the horse, then allow him to cool down in a quiet treatment area.

(2) **Quietly play a tape of pig noises.** Play this at a volume which is sufficiently loud for him to prick his ears, but not so loud as to cause him to become agitated. Stay with him and get him to relax, for example by stroking him gently. Do not switch off the tape until he is fully relaxed. The tape may be restarted and the volume turned up slightly. The process is then repeated. Repeat this several times but do not try too many sessions in one go.

(3) **Repeat stages 1 and 2 using the smell of pigs.** In other sessions the sight of pigs from afar may also be tried in the same way.

(4) **Introduce a pig at increasingly close quarters.** Initially this could be in a nearby stable but should not be so close as to cause anxiety. If it does, then you have tried to do too much too soon. Keep the pig there until he relaxes. When the horse appears to accept the pig at this distance then the pig can be brought nearer the next time. You can continue to work on this as you start from the full distance with stage 5.

(5) **Repeat stage 4, without the preliminary exercise.** As this proves successful, several pigs may be introduced.

This technique can also be used for horses which are difficult to load. In this case the lorry can be left in the field for the horse to become acclimatised to it. Later hay can be placed inside it for the horse to investigate. Then the lorry can be left with the engine running and hay inside. In other sessions the horse can be led towards the lorry without actually being put inside it. Eventually

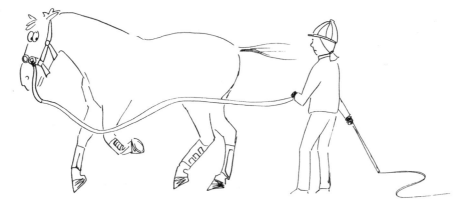

Fig. 9.5 Lungeing a horse before you start a systematic desensitisation programme, will help the horse to relax more deeply during the exposure phase of the treatment.

the horse will accept being loaded; but it should not be transported anywhere until it is very easy to load. It should then be taken on only a short journey and returned to its paddock. If a horse learns that every time it is to be loaded it is going to a show it is likely to get quite excited by the sight of the box, as a result of the process of classical conditioning.

Counterconditioning and overtraining

In this technique the horse is trained to perform a behaviour which is completely incompatible with the one which is to be eliminated. It is used to replace any problem behaviour with another more desirable behaviour and is often combined with systematic desensitisation when treating a fear.

The secret of good counterconditioning is to overtrain the horse before the problem stimulus is introduced. Psychological overtraining (as opposed to physiological overtraining which is a form of over-exercising) involves pairing a stimulus and response so regularly and frequently that the animal responds immediately to the slightest hint of the controlling stimulus. Suppose you have a horse which is scared of the vet, we could use counterconditioning to help relieve this problem.

(1) **The horse is trained that a certain object (say a red handkerchief) means that it must stand still.** This is done by a combination of positive reinforcement and classical conditioning.
(2) **This process is repeated regularly and frequently, for varying lengths of time.** The horse is also trained that when the handkerchief is not present it can fidget about, so if a vet arrives before the programme is complete no handkerchief is displayed.
(3) **When a reliable response has been obtained, a small level of distraction is introduced.** The horse is continuously reinforced for the correct response.
(4) **This process is repeated frequently with increasing levels of distraction.** It is then moved onto an intermittent reinforcement schedule.
(5) **The handkerchief may then be used to get the horse to stand still at any time.**

This process works as long as the association between the handkerchief (stimulus) and the learned response is stronger than the association between any other stimuli in the environment at that time and an alternative response. Many good handlers, who seem to be able to calm a horse simply by their presence, are in fact themselves counterconditioned stimuli for good behaviour.

For safety reasons it is always worth overtraining your horse to stop still in response to a verbal command. This will give you control should you ever get into difficulty. The earlier you start in a horse's development the easier it is to establish overtrained responses.

Join up and follow up

This is a non-confrontational system used for backing and rehabilitating many problem horses. Although round pens have been used for training horses since Roman times, Monty Roberts has popularised the technique in the U.K. and extended its use with a technique which he calls 'Join up'. It is not a difficult skill to develop and is relatively easy to understand in the light of what we have already explained. It simply applies the principles of the three Cs already discussed (communication, co-ordination and cohesion) with the basics of learning theory.

We will describe the 'join-up/follow up' technique here with a brief commentary. Further description and illustration of the technique is available in the text by Bayley and Maxwell given in the reading list at the end of this chapter. Videos of the technique are also available.

(1) **The horse is released into a 15 metre circular pen and encouraged to move round.** This is most easily achieved by throwing a length of lunge line behind the horse. The horse is kept moving at a trot round the outside of the pen, with yourself in the centre. Your body language will encourage him to keep moving: keep your head high and eyes fixed on his and your movements jerky. This will maintain his level of arousal and encourage him to continue avoiding you. The furthest place he can go from you is around the edge.

(2) **After several rounds you should be able to turn him.** This is done by by moving forward from the centre and directly towards his path, as if meeting him face to face. As you enter his flight zone he will naturally turn in order to avoid you. Repeat this procedure several times in order to ensure that you can safely control his behaviour without physical contact.

(3) **After this watch for signs of attention directed towards yourself.** As the horse goes round he will soon realise that there is no escape and so turn to you for some instruction as to what he needs to do in order to get out of this situation. The signs of attention include movement of the inside ear and some bending of the head towards you.

(4) **The horse will then start to 'lick and chew'.** This is probably a displacement reaction caused by the frustration of the situation

(see Chapter 10). When this is combined with a lowering of the head it suggests that the horse is trying to approach. The function of this behaviour is probably similar to the approach gesture of the unsure snapping foal (see Chapter 4).

(5) **The animal now appears willing to accept control of the situation by another.** If you avert your gaze at this point and turn away so that you stand ahead of him at angle of about 45 degrees towards him, he is likely to try and follow. If he moves away, turn suddenly, make eye contact and work him round the pen. He now has a choice for future reference. Either he can approach or he can stay away, in which case there is a price to pay. This is known as response cost punishment and uses the Premack Principle (see above). When he starts to follow, move away from him slowly and smoothly, avoiding eye contact so as not to arouse him.

(6) **As he reaches you, reward him with a gentle stroke.** Continue to avoid eye contact and move towards scratching the withers as he allows. This is 'join up'. He now learns that if he goes with you he is rewarded, otherwise he must work. Move around the pen, turning away from him the whole time, this then gives him the opportunity to follow. If you turn towards him then he has to decide what to do. Should he walk directly at you or turn away? You have given him the initiative and he may make a mistake. This is 'follow up'. Do not follow him if he turns away.

(7) **You should now be able to get him to stand whilst you stroke him and handle him all over.** You should move slowly and smoothly and reassure him as you go. Soon you will be able to introduce a saddle. If he shows any resentment then he is worked around the pen as before with it on until he relaxes. Next a rider may be introduced; he should gradually introduce his weight to the horse and only mount when the horse is able to support the rider's weight laid over his back. Reward for good behaviour is essential.

This technique is not only used for backing horses but also dealing with certain problem horses like those showing some forms of non-fear related aggression. In this case the horse is worked round the pen whenever he shows any aggressive behaviour towards you. It is important that you can safely repel him in these circumstances without injury and the initial ring-work is an essential component of this. It is also important that you feel confident when using these techniques and, if you are in any doubt, that you do not take risks. Consult someone for specialist advice.

Using the flight zone

Working around the edge of a horse's flight zone is a useful way of controlling his behaviour when loose schooling. If you move to stand in front of him and stand at an angle of about 45 degrees towards him you should find that he stops. If you go too far forward he will turn and move away but by stepping in and out of his personal space you should be able to hold him still. When trying to approach a difficult loose horse use a series of approach and avoidance steps. This involves moving towards him, until he shows the first signs of preparing himself to take avoidance action and then stepping out of his flight zone. By repeating this exercise you can soon reduce the size of this area as he learns to accept your proximity.

In order to control a group of loose horses in a field, you only need to be able to identify the controller in the group and then work that animal in this way. The others will stick together as long as you watch your position and technique.

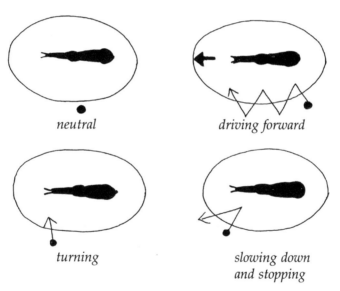

neutral   *driving forward*

turning   *slowing down
and stopping*

Fig. 9.6   Your position relative to the flight zone of the horse may be used to control its movement without other aids.

Conclusion

These techniques involve a simple application of learning principles together with an understanding of horse behaviour. They can be applied in particular contexts in order to create specific treatment protocols according to your own needs. The better your understanding of the principles, the more flexible your approach to problem solving and the better able you will be at dealing with any case. This is why we have avoided prescriptive remedies throughout this text.

TOPICS FOR DISCUSSION

◇ Watch a section of a riding lesson and note the instruction given to the rider to correct the horse's behaviour. Try to describe the associations required for the horse to respond as intended and how these may have been learned.

◇ Behaviourist and cognitive approaches to the study of animal learning are not mutually exclusive but complementary. Discuss.

◇ Consider the stages involved in teaching a horse a new task. Analyse the associations that must be made at each stage and consider how these can be established most efficiently. If possible, try putting this into practice.

◇ Consider situations in which your body language can be used to reinforce the behaviour of a horse whilst it is being schooled.

◇ Discuss situations when it would be preferable to teach a new response through the chaining of several simpler tasks and when it may be preferable to shape a new response.

◇ Consider how we might use counterconditioning to eliminate a certain unwanted behaviour. Draw up a specific treatment schedule for this.

References and further reading

Bayley, L. & Maxwell, R. (1996) *Understanding your Horse*. David & Charles, Newton Abbot.

Chance, P. (1994) *Learning and Behavior*. 3rd edn. Brooks/Cole, Pacific Grove.

Cooper, J.J. (1998) Learning theory and its application in the training of horses. *Equine Veterinary Journal: Behaviour Supplement* (In Press).

Lieberman, D.A. (1993) *Learning, Behavior and Cognition*. 2nd edn. Brooks/Cole, Pacific Grove.

Mills, D.S. (1998) Applying learning theory to the management of the horse: the difference between getting it right and getting it wrong. *Equine Veterinary Journal: Behaviour Supplement* (In Press).

Morgan, C.L. (1894) *An Introduction to Comparative Psychology*. Walter Scott, London.

Premack, D. (1959) Toward empirical behavioural Laws: I. Positive reinforcement. *Psychological Review* **69**, 219–25.

Seligman, M.E.P. (1970) On the generality of the laws of learning. *Psychological Review* **77**, 406–18.

Thorndike, E.L. (1898) Animal intelligence: an experimental study of the associative processes in animals. *Psychological Review, Monograph Supplements* **2** (8), 1–109.

Titchener, E.B. (1896) *A Textbook of Psychology*. Macmillan, New York.

Tolman, E.C. (1932) *Purposive Behaviour in Animals and Man*. Century, New York.

Walker, S. (1987) *Animal Learning, An Introduction*. Routledge & Kegan Paul, London.

Wanless, M., (1995) *Ride with your Mind: A Right Brain Approach to Riding*. Hamlyn, London.

Watson, J.B. (1913) Psychology as the behaviourist views it. *Psychology Review* **20**, 158–77.

Wolpe, J. (1958) *Psychotherapy by Reciprocal Inhibition*. Stamford University Press, Stamford.

10. *Welfare*

Understanding welfare

Everybody who buys a horse wants to look after it and make sure that they look after its well-being. Unfortunately intentions are not always the same as actions. This is not necessarily because we fail to provide what we know every horse needs for its health, like a balanced diet and exercise. Sometimes we just do not know what a horse needs and so do not provide it, or provide what we think is best when this may not be the case.

This section will look at some of these more problematic areas and suggest ways in which we can find out what horses want. We will also look particularly at stereotypic behaviours, or 'vices' as they are commonly known, since they are such a frequent problem.

What is right is not always the same as what is good

Horses were not designed to be ridden. So keeping a horse for riding will always be a compromise between what we want and what we think is fair to do to a horse. This is an ethical decision.

Ethics is concerned with what we should and should not do.

Assessing animal welfare is about finding out how an animal feels about what is happening. We need this information in order to make ethical judgements but we should not confuse the two.

There are certain things which we may think we should never do to a horse, like leave it without water. In which case we can say that horses have certain rights. The law gives horses a number of rights and so the decision about what we should definitely not do is already made; for example, it is illegal to cause unnecessary suffering or to abandon horses. In some situations there is no law to guide us and we must make our own decisions.

We may decide to give horses more rights than they have in law, for example we might consider that every horse has the right to be vaccinated against tetanus and flu. In this case we make sure our horses are regularly vaccinated.

In other situations there is no simple solution that is always right, and so we must make an ethical judgement. For example, if our horse has severe painful arthritis, should we keep him alive? The welfare question is very easy to answer in this situation. Whilst alive he is suffering to some degree, if dead he is not. But his suffering is not the only factor to consider when deciding what is right in this situation. One way to solve this dilemma is to look at the benefits (pros) and costs (cons) of the options and to make a judgement on the basis of which causes most good overall.

This is known as a utilitarian approach to ethical matters. In the example given we would need to ask what are the benefits of keeping our old friend going, like the happiness it brings us to see him each day. Against this we would have to face up to the costs, which include how much he is suffering. The alternative would be 'to call it a day' and to ask the vet to put him down – euthanasia. The benefit in this situation is that he is no longer suffering, the cost is the heartache to us.

Because our own feelings are involved, it is often very difficult for us to make an honest assessment. It is therefore important that we ask and listen to the advice of others, like the vet, who will give us an unbiased and scientific opinion. Whatever conclusion we reach, we should not feel guilty about it because we have done what we think is right given the available facts. If we decide to have him put down it is normal to feel sad and even scared or angry for a while, but that does not mean that we did the wrong thing.

One of the big problems with making this judgement is knowing exactly how much our horse is suffering. This is why the study of animal welfare is so important. If we know what horses do not like or find difficult to cope with, then it is easier to decide what it is right for us to do.

Animal welfare is about finding out the facts. Animal ethics is about judging what is the best thing to do in the light of these facts. Unfortunately there is still an enormous amount that we do not know about what horses need or want and as we shall see, our intuition about this is not necessarily correct.

Measuring welfare

Seeing whether or not your horse is happy.

If we are interested in the study of horse welfare, we are concerned with how a horse feels about things. This is not an easy area of study, as it may lead to misunderstandings about anthropomorphism. If I wanted to know how you felt about something you could tell me and I might believe you. Unfortunately, horses can not talk to us in the same way and so we must use other techniques and measures. When choosing a measure it is important to recognise how that measure relates to the horse's well being. We can look for signs and measures of good welfare and/or poor welfare.

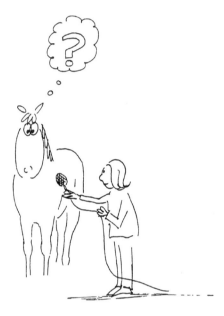

Fig. 10.1   Asking horses directly how they feel does not give us much information.

Good welfare
Measures of good welfare might include:

(1)   A low incidence of disease and injury.
(2)   A good variety of normal behaviours. These include signs of a healthy appetite and normal responsiveness.
(3)   Good performance.

Poor welfare
Measures of poor welfare include:
(1)   **Signs which could lead to suffering if they are not corrected,** e.g.
◇ Changes in the body which make it harder for the horse to fight off disease
◇ Reduced performance
◇ Restriction which does not allow the horse to avoid unpleasant experiences

◇ Changes in character, such as extreme jumpiness or over-cautious behaviour

◇ Behavioural and physiological signs which suggest that the horse has to make quite a significant effort to cope including restlessness.

These signs do not mean that the horse is necessarily suffering at the moment but if they were to continue we might have good reason for concern.

(2) **Signs which indicate that there is an ongoing problem**, e.g.

◇ Sickness, injury and other forms of disease

◇ Behavioural and physiological signs which suggest that the horse is not coping

◇ Fearful behaviour and behaviours associated with attempts to escape from the current situation.

If we see these sorts of sign then we know that the horse has a problem to concern us.

(3) **Signs which suggest that there has been a welfare problem in the past**, e.g.

◇ Severe scars and other deformities as a result of injury and disease

◇ Behavioural scars, i.e. behavioural disturbances that persist even though the cause has gone

◇ Extreme jumpiness, vigilance or apathy.

This description is based on the analysis of Wiepkema and Kool-haas (1993).

Difficulties with the idea of a 'stress hormone'

These measures can be difficult to interpret because there is no universal symptom of poor welfare.

A measure, which may suggest pain in one circumstance, may indicate pleasure in another. For example, the hormone cortisol is released into the blood by the adrenal glands and helps prepare the body to cope when it has to make an effort. The fact that it rises when we would expect the horse to be stressed meant that it came to be known as the 'stress hormone'. Many people thought that if they recorded higher levels than normal this meant the animal was suffering. However, when the body releases this hormone it does not distinguish between the effort that has to be made to cope with something potentially nasty and the effort associated with exploiting pleasurable situations such as mating. This hormone goes up in the same way when a stallion is mating as when he is severely frightened, so this measure is not very specific.

Another problem with cortisol as a measure of suffering is that in some circumstances when we might expect an animal to be suffering, e.g. if the animal is suffering from heat stroke, the level may not rise at all. The cortisol level is therefore inconsistent as a measure of stress. The same can be said of many other physiological measures like the level of reproductive hormones, enzymes and changes in the body like an altered resting heart rate.

Looking at physiological and behavioural measures in context

So what use are these measures?

When we want to work out how an animal is feeling we need to take several measures and look at the context in which the horse finds itself. There is no one single or simple measure of welfare.

Some changes occur in response to an immediate problem. These are acute signs and include:

◇ Increases in heart rate
◇ Increases in respiratory rate
◇ Rises in adrenaline   } (physiological)
◇ Rises in cortisol
◇ Startle reactions (behavioural).

Other changes are only seen if the problem persists, chronic signs like:

◇ Reproductive problems
◇ Gastric ulcers
◇ An increased incidence of disease   } (physiological)
◇ A fall in body weight
◇ The development of unusual behaviours like stereotypies, including weaving, cribbing and windsucking (behavioural).

Interpreting behavioural signs

Some scientists believe that the end point of physiological changes, i.e. the behavioural response, is a more reliable indicator of an animal's quality of life. However the interpretation of these behavioural signs is not without its own difficulties.

For example stereotypies, which are repetitive, relatively invariant behaviours with no apparent function, seem to take some time to develop in response to a welfare problem. This is why we have included them in the list of signs that appear when a problem persists. But once behaviour like weaving has developed, a horse may start to weave as soon as it gets excited or upset. We therefore might include it in the list of signs which occur after there has been a welfare problem.

Another problem with using stereotypic behaviours to assess welfare is understanding what they tell us about a horse's well-being. These sorts of behaviour may help the horse to cope with an unpleasant situation. When a horse is prevented from cribbing it seems to mount a bigger physiological stress response than when it is able to engage in this behaviour.

Although these behaviours only develop when there appears to be a problem with the environment they may then persist even if the horse is provided with everything it could possibly need. Cribbing or any other stereotypic behaviour does not therefore mean that there is currently a problem with its management. It may persist even when previous welfare problems have been sorted out. We will return to this later in the chapter in the section on stereotypies.

Asking horses what they would like

An alternative way to investigate the welfare of a horse is to design experiments to ask a horse what it needs and what it wants. We will first look at the types of experiment that we can do. Then we will look at how we can interpret them and relate them to the well-being of horses.

Studies of natural behaviour

We could look at the behaviour of horses in a rich and unrestricted environment and see how they spend their time and energy. The forces of natural selection mean that horses will spend time and energy on those things which are important to their survival. The difficulty with this approach is that we might be tempted to think that a horse needs to do everything that it does in the wild. There are several problems with this.

(1)   We know that horses get chased and eaten in the wild and that this is not good for them, so there are certainly some 'natural' behaviours which are definitely not necessary for their well-being!

(2)   The wild environment and the domestic one are not the same. Since an animal's behaviour reflects its environment, we would expect its behaviour to be different in the two situations. Differences do not necessarily mean that one is causing problems. Your behaviour on a nice, sunny, all-expenses-paid beach holiday may be very different to your behaviour on a self-catering holiday in Disneyland, but you probably would enjoy both. Differences in behaviour may simply reflect adaptations to different environments.

(3)   There is a difference between the behaviour and the goal. Wild horses spend about 60% of their time grazing because this is the time it takes them to get all the nutrients they need. Many domestic horses are fed special diets, so they can consume a balanced and adequate amount of food in much less time. Is this a problem? It depends on whether there is a need for the behaviour *per se* or only to fulfil the goal of the behaviour. Does a horse need to graze or does it only graze because it needs the nutrients?

Another important question related to this is whether horses need to chew and to have a full stomach in order not to feel hungry. The problem here is whether or not the horse is really well adapted to the environment in which we keep him. Does the domestic environment allow horses to satisfy their essential needs? Horses have adapted to deal with a variety of environments but is the domestic environment a step too far?

Other types of experiment need to be done in order to answer this question, but it does seem that not all things that are natural are necessary. At most, field studies of wild behaviour can simply suggest what is likely to be important to horses.

Simple preference tests

In these experiments we give a horse a choice of environments and see which it prefers. The idea being that it will choose what it is better for it. For example, in a study carried out by Sarah Eckley and supported by the Universities Federation for Animal Welfare we have looked at bedding preferences. We had a two-chamber shelter in which we put two different types of bedding. We then recorded where the horses went. The experiment was repeated several times over a three-month period with different horses and different beddings. We recorded the amount of time spent in each compartment and found that most time was spent on straw and least on paper, wood chip came in between. As a result we could say that the horses preferred straw over wood chip in their stable. But we cannot tell how important straw is in itself to horses. It may be that all three beddings were excellent, but that straw was the best of the three or that all three were poor and straw was the best of a bad lot.

Simple preference tests like this can only tell us how one thing compares to another. But even this is not straightforward. It is rare for every animal in an experiment to make the same exclusive choice. Even if they choose to spend the majority of their time in one particular environment what do we make of their occasional choice of the other environment? It could be that there is still something essential to the animal in this environment, it is just that it does not have to spend much time there in order to achieve what it needs. For example, if we looked at the behaviour of people in their homes we might see that they spent a lot of time in the living room, kitchen and bedroom, but only a small amount of time in the bathroom. However, if for the sake of efficiency we had to eliminate one room in the house, we would not be right to conclude that you could happily do without a bathroom, even though this is the room in which you spend least time. We need therefore to take into account differences in behaviour in the various environments.

Consistent minority choices are common in these tests, because it is normal for an animal to monitor, explore and learn about the whole of the environment available to it. On the other hand we must be aware that this may not be simply investigation of what is there. It may be something more important.

Other problems which we need to appreciate when doing these sorts of test is that animals may initially choose what they are familiar with. For example, when the last pit ponies were brought out of the pits they would prefer to hide away in the dark rather than make use of the open paddocks available to them. With time this changed, but our tests must allow the test subjects to settle and familiarise themselves with the options and consequences of their choice. These problems can be overcome with careful design and even the issues relating to measuring how important something is can be sorted out with sufficient care and forethought.

Preference tests designed to measure how important something is
This can be tested in several ways, but such tests depend on the idea that animals will work harder for the things that are more important to them. Consider the graph in Figure 10.2.

The animal works for the same amount of A no matter what the cost. A may be something like food or water. The fact that the animal does not compromise means that A is an essential commodity. When we increase the cost of product B we find the animal takes less of it. The animal appears to be able to do without it. How

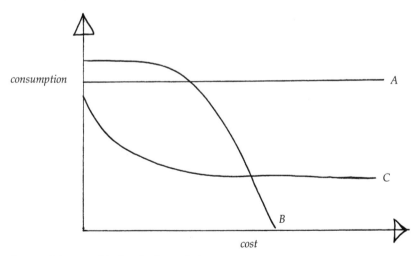

A *essential commodity (e.g. food or water)*
B *luxury (e.g. carrots)*
C *essential, but in less than the preferred quantities (e.g. sweet feed)*

Fig. 10.2 Change in consumption of three commodities with increasing cost.

much the animals initially consume is not important. What is important is how the consumption changes with work required. We can see that whereas the horse will work very hard for A, it will not work very hard for B. B is therefore a luxury of some description, maybe carrots. In graph C, we see demand falling but eventually plateauing out at a certain level. This indicates that C is essential in smaller doses to the horse. It might be a sweet feed.

We could do these experiments with horses with a switch delivering the commodity when the animal has worked for it. We could in theory build a stable with switches controlling the amount of light, the food type, water, space and companionship and then see how the horse arranges things. We could then increase the cost of some of these changes and see how cost affects consumption. The horse's behavioural choices would then tell us how important everything is.

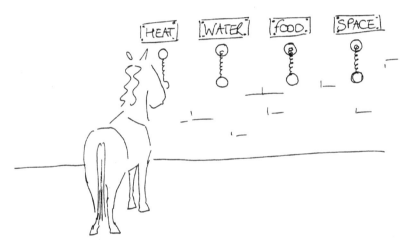

Fig. 10.3 Experiment designed to ask horses what they really want!

The cost which we might impose on an animal in such a system is usually some aspect of work, but other techniques are possible. We might do a simple preference test and then do something to make the preference less attractive. In the example above we could put much brighter lights or excessive heating in the preferred box. We can then see how bright the lights have to be in order for the preference to be reversed. If we cannot reverse the preference without risk of seriously injuring the horse, this would tend to suggest that the requirement is essential to the animal. With sufficient information an animal will only take serious risks for really important things.

A similar but less drastic form of test is to try to trade off one preference against another. For example we could look at the results of the following combinations:

Big box + companion *v* Little box + companion
Big box + no companion *v* Little box + no companion
Big box + companion *v* Little box + no companion
Big box + no companion *v* Little box + companion

These sorts of test help us to establish what an animal's environmental and behavioural priorities are. This way we could establish not only what is essential but also what is important to a horse.

Is the domestic horse a fish out of water?

The behaviour strategies of any animal have evolved because they helped its ancestors adapt to a changing environment. We have looked at the evolutionary history of the horse and so can have some idea of the natural behaviour strategies and priorities which it is likely to have. Domestication may have changed these a little (Chapter 3), but we are likely to see similar behaviour and needs, regulated by similar motivational factors. Selection during domestication is unlikely to have introduced anything radically new.

The captive environment of our pet horse is quite different to that of its wild state. The essentials for life are readily available, and others determine much of what it can do. Apart from deliberate cruelty welfare problems arise for the domestic horse because the strategies and their control mechanisms which have served horses so well in the past are not adequate for the current context. We can illustrate this problem as shown in Figure 10.4.

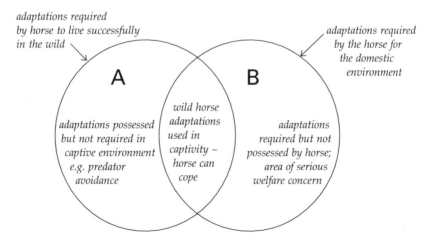

Fig. 10.4 Venn diagram illustrating the relationship between the adaptations possessed by the horse and the demands of living in captivity. The greater the amount of circle B that is contained within circle A, the less the threat to the horse's wellbeing. Adapted from Fraser *et al.* (1997).

Perhaps the two biggest potential problems facing the stabled horse, for which he is not prepared, are how to fill the time available and how to cope with not being in control.

The problem of the time vacuum

Natural selection brings efficiency. The most efficient horses leave more offspring. These are not only the ones with the most efficient behaviour but also the ones which organise their behaviours most efficiently. To be a winner you must stay alive and reproduce as much as possible. The knack is to do these things well and balance the demands of each in the limited time available. So how is the captive environment different? Let us look more closely.

Our typical domestic horse is provided with a balanced diet and water in a readily available form. It is protected from the elements in the security and confinement of a stable. This means it can only really take exercise when we say so. Breeding also tends to be controlled and condensed into as short a time as possible. So those activities that the horse has probably evolved to value highly have been met in relatively little time. But there are still 24 hours in the day so what does the horse do?

Now it seems that behaviours which can expand to fill the time may be essential for the horse's well-being. When there is limited time available, these behaviours are not a priority as they are not essential to keeping the animal alive. The most obvious natural behaviours which serve this purpose are play and investigatory behaviour. We see these in wild horses when times are good, but play and investigation, which are not directed to finding something which might keep the horse alive, soon disappear when times are hard. Why should these behaviours be so important when life is easy? Probably because they not only pass the time of day but allow the animal to learn more about its environment and so be better prepared for when times are hard again. Horses which did not explore their environment might have been more likely to fall prey to predators and did not know as much about the game of life as the others when times got hard again. The tendency to play and explore was then an adaptive trait which was not selected against and so still exist in the horse today.

The problem for the domestic horse is not how to achieve its needs, dropping non-essentials when times are hard, but how to fill the time available with the limited number of behaviours at his disposal (Figure 10.5).

Whether or not a lack of things to do causes the feeling of boredom in the horse, we do not know. An alternative explanation might propose that horses which rested when times are easy, might

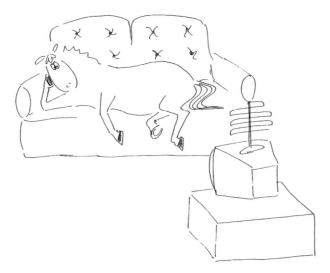

Fig. 10.5 One of the problems for the captive horse may be how to fill the day with the behaviours available.

have conserved energy better for the harder times. In which case it would have been adaptive for horses to just stand dozing when they have met their essential needs. Horses are individuals and some, even when in an environment where there are opportunities for play and investigation, do not indulge in these activities. However it seems that as you meet the essential needs of an animal, some of the luxuries become more important for its well being. Depriving any animal of something for which it is willing to make an extreme effort is not good for its welfare and this may apply to apparent luxuries in the domestic situation.

The practical point of all this is that we should make sure that horses in the stable for long periods have several suitable ways other than sleep to fill the time of day. Otherwise our horse may suffer and we can expect problems.

Not being in control

Being in control seems to be an important part of reducing stress. Contrary to popular belief it is not so much the top high-flying executives who suffer from stress but more those people who are working their way up and do not know whether or not they will make it, and those who face job insecurity. This also seems to apply to animals. Lack of control may therefore present a welfare problem in its own right and it may also give rise to specific welfare concerns. The domestic horse has problems with being out of control on two important fronts:

(1)   His life is controlled by others to such a degree that he may get frustrated because he cannot get what he needs when he needs it.
(2)   The mechanisms designed to control certain behaviours are no longer appropriate because the goal is achieved in a different way.

We will discuss each of these in turn.

Not having what you want when you want it

As caring owners it is normal to want to provide what is best for our horses. We provide food and fresh water and shelter. A good stable keeps your horse in and provides shelter and comfort in bad weather. It not only protects your horse but also keeps him clean. However stable design seems to be important in influencing the development of some problems. Your horse is kept in the stable until you let him out and he is limited in what he can do when he is here.

Think about when you feed him. You prepare the meal and bring it to him. Even if he is the only horse on the yard, he will detect the signs that he is about to be fed. This excites him. All the signs of food are there but he cannot get to it yet. This may be the highlight of his day indoors and so all the systems kick in to get him ready for food. Although he does eventually get his food, this regular cycle of excitement and delay may be very frustrating to him. This, it is thought, may lead to a number of problems.

Perhaps the simplest and most obvious is troublesome behaviour in the stable. If you feed him while he is kicking the door in excitement, learning theory (see Chapter 9) predicts that he will be more likely to do it in future when he is similarly aroused. We then end up with a horse that bangs the door at feed times.

It is surprising how many behaviours can be conditioned in this way. Stable fed horses often appear to develop rituals or apparently superstitious behaviour patterns at feeding time, e.g. they may circle before they feed. Such behaviours have probably been conditioned as a result of the reward of feeding. They just happened to be doing it when the food finally arrived and so associate the two.

This is not the only frustration for the horse in a stable. It may get excited at the prospect of going out but has to wait until you have put its rugs or tack on. The evolution of the horse has not designed it to wait when it wants something. They are animals of the great outdoors in control of their own lives that do things when it suits them. They flee now, and find out later; so they may not have the mechanisms in place to allow them patiently to wait their turn.

We just do not know how good horses are at coping with this

problem, but we do know that a number of aspects of life in a stable seem to be associated with behavioural problems. Some, like stereotypic behaviour (see below) may not simply be learned problems but a sign of a more fundamental mental disturbance or illness.

'I've started but I can't finish'

Other frustrations associated simply with stable design include that of social contact. Horses seem to have a strong tendency to seek social contact and for this reason it is generally not recommended to keep a horse on a yard on its own, but to provide some form of companion. However, even if there are other horses on the yard, as long as our horse is in the stable he cannot touch or interact with them in the normal equine way and this could be terribly frustrating. All the cues are there for social interaction, they can call to each other, they can see, hear and smell each other, but they cannot complete the social ritual. Whether or not horses feel a sense of mental frustration, we can be sure that this represents a form of behavioural frustration. We should not be surprised, therefore, when problems develop. For much of the day the horse could be starting behaviour patterns that he cannot complete.

Goals too easily satisfied

We saw earlier how behaviour was motivated and regulated by its own consequences. This regulatory system has developed to be efficient in a natural setting where certain associations have been reliable for millions of years. For example, horses have been obtaining their daily requirement of energy from grass for this length of time. Grass varies from place to place and time to time and there is no advantage in eating a lot more than is necessary. It just makes the horse overweight and easy meat for predators. So how does the body know that it has had enough?

It seems that the body depends on a number of signals which indicate that the horse has had sufficient. This includes how much it has chewed, how full its stomach is, how long it is since it last ate anything, how active it has been and what effect the food is having on its blood sugar levels and in the gut. The brain then makes a decision telling the horse in the wild to stop on the basis of this overall picture.

So what might happen to our domestic horse that has his food available as concentrates and high quality grass? These do not need as much chewing nor do they fill the gut as much as the food that horses are adapted to eat. As a result, although you have met his physiological requirements in order for him to maintain his weight, his brain does not recognise this; he is still driven to chew. The result might be a horse which eats too much for his size, a horse that eats his bedding, a horse that chews wood or possibly even cribs and wind-sucks (see below), just so that he can satisfy his hunger.

For a long time scientists have been unsure whether animals need to carry out certain behaviours or whether they simply need to satisfy the goals of these behaviours. If animals have behavioural needs then preventing any of these behaviours is likely to cause welfare problems. If, on the other hand, animals need only the goals of the behaviours, then we can satisfy their requirements by making sure we supply all these goals. In the example above, we are suggesting a compromise. In order to satisfy a need it may be necessary to satisfy the mechanisms which govern its expression. These may include certain elements of the behaviour alone, with or without a wide range of internal physiological processes which go beyond the obvious goal of the behaviour. For horses in nature the goal, the physiological processes and the behaviour have always gone together, but in the captive environment man has pulled them apart. As a result we may get problems. One question, which is unlikely to be answered for a long time, is what conscious feelings are involved with each decision.

Stereotypies

Stereotypies are repetitive behaviours which do not seem to vary much but have no obvious function. It includes the following behaviours:

(1) **Cribbing or crib-biting** The horse repeatedly grabs something (often the top of a stable door or feed manger) with its front teeth, arches its neck and usually grunts as it pulls back and lets go.
(2) **Weaving** The horse repeatedly shifts his weight from one side to the other. The head and neck are usually swung at the same time and the feet lifted of the ground in the same order as occurs when he is walking.
(3) **Wind-sucking** The horse appears to gulp air repetitively. A grunt usually accompanies the effort, but recent research suggests very little air, if any, is actually swallowed. Cribbing often occurs in the same horse.

The list could also include box-walking and compulsive wood-chewing and other unusual behaviours like tongue-lolling. Other behaviours are fixed but not particularly repetitive, like star-gazing. In this situation the horse suddenly freezes and turns his head up; he then just stands there apparently oblivious to the world.

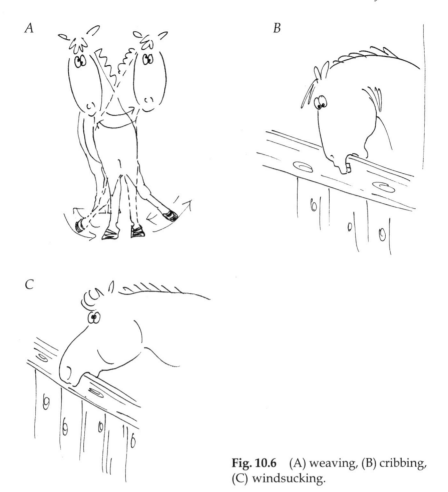

Fig. 10.6   (A) weaving, (B) cribbing, (C) windsucking.

Obsessive compulsive disorders or stable vices?

Partly because some of these behaviours do not really fit into the definition given above for a stereotypy and since some of the classic stereotypies can be quite variable, some authors have described them all as obsessive-compulsive disorders or OCDs (Luescher *et al.*, 1991). This term was chosen because they look like the signs of the human mental disorder of the same name. There are several potentially serious problems with this definition though.

(1)   **The term OCD is a diagnostic term.** This means that it implies something about what is happening inside the horse's head (see Chapter 1). From the point of view of describing behaviour it is useful to have a term which describes the behaviour before we try to describe the motivation behind the behaviour. So the term OCD does not help us in this respect.

(2)   **Are horses obsessive?** If an animal has an OCD, we are saying

it has an obsession and a compulsion. An obsession is a persistent thought which underlies the process. We do not know what horses think so this description is a guess at the unknown The 'obsessive' part of the term does not add much to the definition bringing only an unnecessary anthropormorphic complication. The term compulsion means that the animal performs the behaviour persistently, and this description is more appropriate as we can see that the animal still tries to continue with the behaviour when we make it much harder for it to do so.

(3) **The term OCD implies that all of these behaviours have a common cause.** By using a diagnostic term for all of these behaviours, we are implying that they are all the same disorder, which is based in anxiety. This idea that there may be a single cause for these behaviours is held by even some of the scientists who prefer the term 'stereotypy'. However, repetitive behaviours occur in many other human diseases including schizophrenia and autism, so why should we assume one common cause for the behaviours in other animals. The evidence does not support this. Some may not even be diseases at all but simply learned stimulus–response habits. Stereotypies are more likely to be similar signs of a wide range of conditions.

For these reasons we will avoid using the term OCD to describe these behaviours although some, but not all, may represent this sort of disorder. Applied animal behaviour science encounters many of these terminological confusions and so it is important to be clear about what you mean when you use a given term.

Any behaviour that an owner does not like may be referred to as a vice. This term is also misleading, as it may suggest that there is something morally wrong with the horse. Although horses may perform behaviours which we do not like, this does not mean that it is their fault, rather it may be a product of the environment. It may be that, by using such a term as 'stable vices', people have been able to justify some pretty cruel treatments for their control, like the use of spiked collars. Equally the extremes which people will go to in order to try and control these behaviours suggest that they are a big concern for owners. Anyway for the purpose of this text we will use the term stereotypic behaviours or stereotypies.

What are stereotypies a sign of?

This question has bothered scientists for a long time. In fact it still bothers many of us. Stereotypic behaviours are common in domestic animals but have not been reported in animals that have never been kept in captivity. It seems that something between 5% and 20% of horses on any given yard may show one or more of these behaviours (McGreevy *et al.*, 1995a). They are therefore a fairly common behaviour in captivity which we do not see in the wild. It also seems that there is a difference in the form and control of these behaviours as they develop. For this reason it is useful to distinguish three separate but similar behavioural situations:

(1) **Behaviours which are repeated several times because of the recurrence or continued presence of their cause** For example, if we isolate a mare from her foal, in a box, it is normal for the mare to paw at the ground repeatedly. She may continue to do so until reunited with her foal. We have already explained earlier in this chapter, how some horses may develop bizarre behaviours and rituals around the time of feeding as a result of reinforcement and these will recur whenever there is the prospect of food. When an animal performs these behaviours it still appears to be aware of its environment and capable of responding to new cues which are significant. The behaviour is also quite variable in its form as it is directly associated with changes in the environment.

(2) **Behaviours which have become stereotyped (early stage stereotypies)** When a behaviour is repeated many times to a similar stimulus, it starts to become streamlined and is more easily triggered by such stimuli. Streamlining means the rough edges get knocked off and the behaviour becomes more consistent in its form. Imagine you are trying to improve your tennis serve. You practice throwing the ball to a particular height and swinging your racket to make the best possible contact. Initially, you are not very good and only occasionally make a good serve, but, as you practice, your behaviour changes and you make good serves more often. Although rewards may speed up the process, they are not necessary and this behaviour may develop simply as a stimulus–response habit without a reward, as a result of sensitisation of the appropriate neural pathways (see Chapter 5). This law of learning was first described by Guthrie (1935) and is like the overtraining exercises described earlier (Chapter 9). Whilst science has moved on in many ways and the explanations and implications of Guthrie's work have changed from his day, this behavioural phenomenon remains a valid observation. It also seems that the process of getting closer to your goal provides its own reinforcement. At this point we have behaviours which are fairly fixed in their form and easily released by specific stimuli.

(3) **Established stereotypies (late stage stereotypies)** With time it seems that stereotypies may no longer be triggered by specific stimuli but may be expressed whenever the animal reaches a certain level of arousal or even spontaneously. The behaviour is then said to have become 'emancipated' from its original cause. At this point

a change in the environment will not bring about a change in the behaviour. It remains as a scar of what has gone on before.

This classification helps to explain, at least in part why treating these behaviours can be so difficult. A thorough case history and careful observations are essential if we are to stand any hope of distinguishing between these behaviours which may look very similar. It also seems that the regulation of the behaviour is different involving different nervous pathways and regions of the brain. Failure to distinguish any such categories of behaviour will, at best, result in inconsistent results; and this is very common in the scientific literature. If a behaviour occurs repeatedly over time we may see the changes described above. In this case, the next question we need to answer is what causes a behaviour to be repeated so frequently. This is discussed in the next section.

What causes stereotypy?

We are now concerned with identifying the factors which lead to the performance of repetitive behaviour, through its development and on to emancipation. We will also consider why these factors should be more common in the domestic environment. Again, there are several explanations, any of which may theoretically be appropriate for any given case. The behaviour may result from learning, frustration or lack of things to do, or be a result of a genuine disease. Each of these will be discussed below.

Learned generalisation to a wider range of stimuli

Imagine we train a horse (intentionally or otherwise) to respond to a certain type of stimulus and continue to reward it for responding to a wide range of stimuli. Stimulus discrimination will not occur as this is not possible. In fact, under these conditions, the behaviour starts to occur to an even wider range of stimuli, a phenomenon known as 'stimulus generalisation'. It will then recur more frequently simply because there are a wider range of stimuli which trigger it even if we remove the reinforcement.

Suppose we are preparing our horse's daily feed. He may get excited in anticipation of what is going to happen as he sees you arrive and go to the feed room. He may even pace on the spot as an expression of this excitement. What happens then? Well, depending on where his stable is in relation to the other horses, he will get fed sooner or later. It may well be that in this situation we are unintentionally conditioning him to perform the behavioural basis (Stage 1) of weaving. He is then rewarded for weaving at least once a day. Since behavioural Stage 1 weaving (as opposed to stereotypic weaving) when you appear has been rewarded, he may be more likely to engage in this sort of behaviour whenever you appear. You may not feed him every time but are likely at least to say 'hello'. Now imagine, the yard is fairly quiet during the day, what does your social contact mean to your horse? It is a reward. So now he weaves whenever you appear. Weaving is now starting to occur in a wider range of situations. In fact as there is so little other excitement on the yard, the level of general arousal may become classically conditioned to the specific motivational factors. The horse now weaves whenever there is any excitement, no matter what the cause. As the behaviour is repeated and this association reinforced, the specific motivational factors become increasingly unnecessary. We then have a horse that weaves for ever increasing periods.

Frustration

We saw in Chapter 5 that a behavioural response occurs as a result of the interaction of both general and specific motivational factors. We also distinguished between appetitive and consummatory behaviours and their feedback effects on the motivational state of the individual. Appetitive behaviours tend to encourage further behaviour towards the goal. When consumption is possible, it appears to initially encourage further persistence, but eventually both the behaviour and its consequences seem to inhibit further consummatory behaviour. The consequences of consummatory behaviour include the effect that consumption has on a number of physiological receptors designed to limit intake. Now let us consider a couple of situations that arise in the domestic situation where this system might get into trouble.

Problems can arise where a horse can see but cannot touch the goal. For example a horse in a stable is unable to complete a close social greeting ritual with another horse opposite which he can see, smell and call to. The horse is highly motivated to engage in closer social behaviour but is physically unable to do so because of the confinement of the stables. We can assume that the sight, smell and sound of another horse are powerful stimuli which lead to the appetitive phase. What then happens? The horse gets stuck in the appetitive phase, i.e. he keeps trying to do the behaviours which would normally lead to the goal. This might involve frustrated attempts at trying to walk towards his partner. Since this is an insoluble problem, we can see him getting caught in a 'continuous loop' of appetitive behaviour until something else intervenes. This situation then creates the perfect environment for progression from Stages 1 to 3 described above. Theoretically we may then end up with a horse which weaves at its door.

As an alternative to a repetition of the appetitive behaviour, we may see behaviours associated with the frustration. These may be a redirected form of the behaviour, a displacement reaction, ambivalent behaviour or some expression of aggression.

(1) **Redirected behaviour** is the normal response to a stimulus directed at something other than the normal goal because this is unreachable. In this case the horse may walk round its box because it is unable to walk across the yard. The result may then be a repetitive and ultimately stereotypic box-walker. This compensates for the frustration of the real goal.

(2) **A displacement behaviour** is an apparently pointless or irrelevant behaviour which occurs when an ongoing activity is thwarted. This may be because the frustration of one behaviour removes the inhibition on other behaviours. This inhibition is important in normal circumstances as it stops us trying to do too many things at once. Perhaps the most commonly seen displacement behaviour seen in the horse is eating. We may then have the setting for developing a compulsive wood-chewer.

(3) **An ambivalent behaviour** is a sequence of actions which contain parts of two different, often opposite behaviours either simultaneously or alternately. It can be described in another way in the terms of a 'should I or shouldn't I?' behavioural dilemma. In this case, it may be that the horse turns away from its companion and then immediately turns back. Once again, this is a potential recipe for weaving.

(4) **Aggressive behaviour** is another common manifestation of frustration and associated with its emotional impact. In our horse it might be expressed directly, for example as door kicking. Alternatively it may be redirected, and it is possible that wood-chewing, wind-sucking and or cribbing are some-times redirected forms of oral aggression.

These states will continue until something intervenes. That something could be one of two situations.

The horse is given access to the goal or a suitable substitute. In which case the behaviours are likely to be reinforced and likely to recur in future.

Alternatively, another behaviour may become a priority. The speed with which this occurs will depend on the rate of the increase in specific motivation for something else or of the fall in motivation for the ongoing behaviour. Remember, the expression of a behaviour may result from its own motivation or from a fall in the motivation for something else (see Figure 5.12). Other behaviours which may intervene as a result of their own specific motivational accumulation and so overtake the ongoing frustrated behaviour include eating and drinking. Moreover, if the goal of the frustration is removed, i.e. the other horse disappears, the motivation for the frustrated behaviour is likely to fall and so other behaviours can be expressed more readily. A similar example could be given for the sight of a field and the frustration of exercise.

Now let us consider another example. The sight, smell and other signs of food may encourage all sorts of appetitive oral feeding behaviours which the horse may find can be satisfied until the arrival of the food by chewing wood. When the food arrives, we have a double reward for wood-chewing. It was satisfying in itself and also led to the best meal of the day! Frustration and reinforcement are then both involved in encouraging the further development of the behaviour into a stereotypy.

There are also problems where the goal is not satisfying enough of itself. Let us suppose we feed our horse a highly concentrated diet. Although this provides him with all the nutrients that he needs, his feeding requirement was not designed to be regulated by nutrient intake, but by the rules of thumb which predict nutrient intake. We then have the situation described in the section 'Goals too easily satisfied' above.

In this situation the goal is provided sooner rather than later and so we do not develop a problem from the frustration of appetitive behaviour. However, because the goal is not in a natural form, the normal process of feedback, relating to the control of consummatory behaviour, does not return the horse to a satisfied state.

Repeated attempts may then be made to produce sufficient feedback to halt the consummatory process. If an effective strategy is found then it will be used whenever necessary. It may be that cribbing, wood-chewing and wind-sucking are in fact substitutes for those parts of the normal eating process which lead to the cessation of feeding. The work of Ralston and his colleagues (Ralston, 1984) suggests that oro–pharyngeal signals are more important than gastro–intestinal ones for the regulation of food intake in the horse. Similarly, weaving and box walking may be substitutes for an endogenous exercise requirement or locomotory goal.

Whether a behaviour acts as compensation for a frustrated appetitive behaviour or substitute for the consummatory behaviour, it is likely that it will be less effective than the real thing at providing feedback. As a result the animal needs to do more of it, in order to get the same level of feedback. This requirement for more of the behaviour may itself put in place the conditions for its further development into a stereotypy.

Behaviour to fill the day and make you feel better

We have already suggested that one of the problems facing the domestic horse is that it has a limited range of behaviours that it can use to fill the day in a stable. It may be that stereotypies or their precursors originate as novel time filling behaviours. Because there is so much time to fill these behaviours are then performed very frequently and for long periods of time. Some of these stereotypies, like wind-sucking are rather bizarre, so why should horses perform such behaviours in preference to more normal ones?

One explanation may be that the performance of some stereotypies is associated with the release of the body's natural painkillers (endorphins and enkephalins) which can make you feel a lot happier. Accordingly it has been suggested that animals may stereotype to help themselves to cope with the environment. This may be appropriate when there is little else to do or when the horse is acutely frustrated as in the situations described, above. If you remove all the surfaces on which a cribbing horse can crib, then we see a lot of physiological changes which might be interpreted as increased stress and a greater effort to cope (McGreevy & Nicol, 1995). Whether or not horses primarily stereotype in order to gain this reward, it is important to remember, when considering the implications of different treatments for these conditions, that physical prevention seems to cause further welfare problems.

Primary pathology

So far all of the explanations for the development of stereotyped behaviour have described a progressive situation. Some behaviours which appear to be stereotyped seem to occur in the final stage spontaneously. These are more likely to be indicative of a physical disease state. This suspicion always arises in conditions where the behaviour appears to be independent of environmental influences.

From this, it may be inferred that late stage stereotypies represent some form of psychological disease. This may be true, as people in a state of chronic anxiety may develop obsessive compulsive disorders. Other psychological illnesses that may be an appropriate model for different stereotyping individuals include schizophrenia and autism.

However, some stereotypies may be signs of primary systemic diseases. Head-shaking can at the most simple level be a normal response to flies or a sign of excitement, but it may also be a sign of disease if the horse throws its head up and down persistently for no apparent reason. In some cases this may be a stereotypic development of the normal behaviour, but more often there is a clearer medical cause. Cook in 1980 listed around 58 causes of persistent head-shaking, which included a range of conditions from allergies to food and pollen, reactions to pain and diseases of the nerves, ear and eye. But even this list is not exhaustive, as it did not include a range of potentially significant middle ear diseases or mental disorders. If any of these conditions is left untreated the behaviour could develop into a persistent stereotypy, which remains even after the cause is gone. It is perhaps not surprising therefore that many cases of head-shaking remain undiagnosed and untreated and that owners turn to alternative therapies in the hope of a cure.

Reducing the risk of stereotypies

Risk factors

It is impossible to give a single cause for stereotyped behaviour. Indeed it is impossible to give a single cause for one type of stereotypy since the behaviour is the final common pathway of many conditions.

A stereotypy is a sign not a diagnosis. In this regard it is similar to the circumstances of feeling sick whilst travelling on a ship. There are many reasons why you might feel sick in this situation – it may be because of the rough seas, or it may be because of something you ate, or maybe you had too much to drink the previous night, etc. Equally we must be aware of the possibility that it is a combination of such factors.

Successful treatment involves addressing all the causal factors, but there is no recipe for success in every case. Not all the horses in a given environment develop stereotypies and there is evidence to suggest that the tendency to perform certain stereotypies may be heritable (Vecchiotti & Galanti, 1986). This would imply that genetic factors might be important. However, genetic inheritance, like the other factors discussed above, is not a cause of stereotypies, but rather a contributing risk factor. With our current knowledge, prevention and treatment should be focussed on reducing as many such factors as possible.

Specific effects of certain factors

McGreevy *et al.* (1995b) found that various factors were associated with an increased reported risk of the following group of behaviours: weaving, box-walking, crib-biting, wind-sucking and wood-chewing. These were:

◇ less than 6.8 kg of forage per day
◇ bedding types other than straw
◇ yards with less than 75 horses
◇ boxes which minimised social contact between neighbouring horses
◇ the use of hay as the source of forage
◇ offering forage more than three times a day
◇ the absence of a paddock on the yard.

More specifically the use of bedding types other than straw particularly affected the amount of weaving, whilst the lower level of
forage specifically seemed to affect the amount of wood-chewing
and weaving.

Redbo *et al.* (1998) have studied the same behaviours in populations of Standardbred trotters and Thoroughbred flat racers. They
found stereotypies other than wood-chewing to be more common
amongst the Thoroughbred population. This population also had
less social contact with companions, less free time outside the
stable, longer training periods and more concentrate in their diet.

When each population was examined separately it was found
that smaller amounts of roughage were related to an increased risk
of wood-chewing in both populations. The other behaviours were
associated with specific risk factors amongst the Thoroughbred
population. Here, the amount of concentrate, the amount of
roughage and the number of horses per trainer were all significantly
related to the occurrence of stereotypic behaviour.

It seems from current ongoing research that the method of
weaning appears to influence the type of stereotypy shown. Foals
which are individually boxed are apparently more likely to become
box-walkers and weavers, whilst group weaned foals may be more
prone to oral stereotypies. This might be because box weaned foals
tend to show more locomotory activity, whilst group weaned
individuals show more suckling-type behaviour. In these cases
stereotypy expression later in life may be a consequence of some
form of psychological regression to the behaviours associated with
stress early in life. This is not surprising if we consider how the
nervous system and behavioural tendencies are moulded by early
experience in so many other ways (see Chapter 4).

Avoidance of risk factors is not a guarantee of success in prevention since there are inevitably more that we do not know about.
Also some of the factors identified above may not themselves be the
problem but co-incidentally identified since they correlate with it.
For example, McGreevy *et al.* found smaller yards to be associated
with a higher risk of problems. This risk may relate to the level of
activity on the yard through the day or some other management
factor. We just do not know what is the really important part of this
correlation. A similar problem exists in all complex factors which
are correlated with a risk.

Principles of treatment for stereotypies and other behaviour problems

By now it should be apparent that it is pointless to produce a list of
specific treatments and their pros and cons. The control of

behaviour is too complicated for that. There is also an ever-increasing range of products on the market. Take professional advice and consider the implications of what is being recommended. Anybody offering a treatment based on scientific principles should also be able to explain how it is likely to work. The purpose of treatment is to make the horse better. It is therefore important to appreciate as far as possible the welfare implications of both the problem behaviour and the possible treatments. In some circumstances it is preferable to leave the horse alone and just to accept the behaviour.

Behaviour may relate to welfare in one of four ways:

(1) It may be a sign of poor welfare, e.g. the depressed stance adopted by a sick horse.
(2) It may indicate the measures which must be taken in order for the animal to adapt to its environment, e.g. some forms of wood-chewing may be a form of roughage supplementation.
(3) It may cause harm or injury, e.g. self-mutilation.
(4) It may be incidental to the animal's well-being, e.g. playing with a fitting in the stable.

The first stage of treatment is to recognise these possibilities and ensure no harm is done. A vet should be consulted in order to rule out disease. A number of strategies are then available for treatment.

(1) The behaviour can be prevented from being expressed.
(2) The causes can be removed.
(3) The animal's perception of its environment can be changed.
(4) The problem behaviour can be redirected onto a non-problem area.
(5) Other behaviours can be encouraged in order to compete with and suppress the expression of the problem behaviour.

These strategies may be implemented using the following techniques:

◇ Applying specific training and psychotherapy techniques
◇ Altering the environment
◇ Using chemical agents like drugs and food supplements to change the behaviour
◇ Using surgery.

We will now consider the implications of each strategy for the welfare of the horse. The strategy used is generally of more importance for the well-being of the horse than the technique, but any intervention carries its own specific risks. These must be evaluated before any treatment offered.

Preventing the behaviour

Prevention is used quite a lot in the management of behaviour problems. It also takes many forms: from isolating the horse that is aggressive to others or muzzling the crib-biter (both forms of environmental manipulation) to the sedation of the horse which is difficult to clip and the surgical removal of the nerves and muscles associated with the act of crib-biting (modified Forsell's operation). These techniques vary in their effectiveness, e.g. many horses still weave behind weaving bars.

Other treatments may be more effective at eliminating the problem but they still do not address the underlying causes. In fact they may make the psychological situation worse. We have already seen how the prevention of cribbing seems to cause further stress. Such changes may also reduce the horse's ability to adapt and respond to other more useful long-term treatments.

In the short term when there is a risk of harm, for example in the aggressive horse, prevention by environmental control is often quick and effective. It may then be a useful stop-gap to prevent further harm until other measures take effect.

It has also been suggested that in the case of established stereotypic behaviours, prevention may be an essential part of an holistic treatment regime. These behaviours may be a special case because they may persist even after the causal factors are removed. Other behaviours should also be encouraged at this time, in order to direct the treatment along safe lines.

Removing the cause of the problem

This is often considered the ultimate objective of a treatment programme but it is not always possible. Sometimes we just do not know what the cause of a problem is, and so are unable to remove it.

If a horse is aggressive because it is a rig or has an ovarian tumour, surgery is the treatment of choice. A mare who persistently rubs her tail may have a pin worm infection which can be treated by anthelmintic drugs.

The presence of resident mares at a stud may sometimes cause increased aggressive competition between stallions. Removing the mares in this case is an effective environmental treatment of the cause of the problem.

The removal of attention that might reinforce an attention-seeking behaviour, like door banging, is an effective psychological intervention for this particular problem.

Changing the patient's perception

If an orphan foal is to be adopted by a mare who has lost her own foal, the use of amniotic fluids familiar to the mare may change her perception of the foal so that it is more readily accepted. Other measures include sprays to block the mare's sense of smell and the use of the dead foal's skin. These traditional techniques all work by altering the mare's perception of her new charge.

The most commonly used psychological technique which fits into this category is systematic desensitisation ((see Chapter 9). This technique is widely used and extremely effective in the treatment of fears, phobias and over-excited responses to certain stimuli. An alternative technique is the use of flooding for the management of these conditions. It might also be argued that anti-anxiety drugs or feed supplements like tryptophan also work at this level as they do nothing to address the fundamental cause but eliminate the problem associated with the perception of a poor environment.

When these techniques are used effectively to address a behaviour that is of welfare concern, then the immediate concern is resolved but the fundamental cause remains. For example, anti-anxiety medication may be used to treat certain forms of stereotyped behaviour in the early stages of their development. The behaviour problem in these cases is usually a result of the management conditions. Anxiolytics may eliminate the anxiety underlying the development of the stereotypy but they do not change the management and design of the yard. These factors should be addressed in the longer term whilst the drugs are used as an immediate stop-gap.

Redirection of the behaviour
If we redirect a problem behaviour away from a problem area towards an acceptable one, then the welfare of the performer remains unchanged (unless he was previously harming himself) but the stress on the owner is reduced. This technique is most commonly used with wood-chewing or cribbing, when the horse is trained to use a suitable board which can be replaced easily. A rubber cribbing board prevents wear of the teeth and a wooden panel meets the needs of the horse without the destruction of the stable. When using such measures it is important to combine them with appropriate training to encourage use of the new focus for attention.

Cribbing can be a very distressing behaviour for owners and can lead them to seek extreme measures for its control. If treatment of the underlying cause is not possible or successful, this technique is preferable to those aimed at prevention, for the reasons already discussed. Its success may depend on not only persuading the horse to use it but also the owner. This is usually possible when a careful explanation of the situation is given.

Increasing behavioural competition
An alternative to redirecting behaviour is to substitute it for another more acceptable one. The ease with which this can be achieved will

depend on the relative strengths of motivation for the competing behaviours. If we introduce toys or food balls for horses in a stable, these may provide the horse with an alternative behaviour to the problem one, but what is the incentive for change? This is where training may help. The horse should be encouraged to use the new toy and, when this appears to be acceptable to it, discouraging the problem behaviour may begin through the careful use of punishment.

We must be careful about checking the acceptability to horses of toys which seem fine to us. Some toys may in fact increase frustration and they will then make matters worse.

Behavioural competition may also be introduced through the process of counter-conditioning (see Chapter 9). As long as the horse still has the opportunity to perform the problem behaviour but chooses not to as a result of encouragement towards other activities, it is likely to be better off as a result of treatment.

Conclusion

When trying to decide how to treat a behaviour problem, try to consider why the horse is performing in this way. Consider the options for treatment, their benefits and risks. Try then to balance this against the effects of doing nothing. We should avoid the tendency to rush and try to eliminate the behaviour at any cost, because we ourselves find it annoying or disturbing. By learning more about equine science we can have greater confidence that our well-meaning intentions towards the horse translate into its improved well-being. This is one of the greatest prizes science can offer.

TOPICS FOR DISCUSSION

◇ Consider the ethical arguments for and against the use of horses for riding.

◇ Discuss the problems associated with measuring the 'feelings' of a horse. What methods might we use to examine this issue?

◇ Consider the treatments available for the control of a range of equine behaviour problems. What strategy does each use to achieve its goal and what is the likely impact of this on the well-being of the horse?

◇ Discuss the pros and cons of preference tests for assessing what a horse really wants.

◇ Discuss what should be considered the main welfare concerns relating to horses in this country today.

◇ Consider what practical measures could be taken to improve the well-being of horses on a yard of your choice.

References and further reading

Barnard, C.J. & Hurts, J.L. (1996) Welfare by design: The natural selection of welfare criteria. *Animal Welfare* **5**, 405–33.

Cook, W.R. (1980) Headshaking in horses Part 4: Special diagnostic procedures. *Veterinary Medicine, Equine Practice* **2** (2), 7–15.

Fraser, D., Weary, D.M., Pajor, E.A. & Milligan, B.N. (1997) A scientific conception of animal welfare that reflects ethical concerns. *Animal Welfare* **6**, 187–205.

Guthrie, E.R. (1935) *The Psychology of Learning*. Harper & Row, New York.

Kiley-Worthington, M. (1997) *Equine Welfare*. J.A. Allen, London.

Lawrence, A.B. & Rushen, J. (eds) (1993) *Stereotypic Animal Behaviour: Fundamentals and Application to Animal Welfare*. CAB International, Wallingford.

Luescher, U.A., McKeown, D.B. & Halip, J. (1991) Reviewing the causes of obsessive-compulsive disorders in horses. *Veterinary Medicine, Equine Practice* **86** (5), 527–30.

Mason, G. (1991) Stereotypies: a critical review. *Animal Behaviour* **41**, 1015–37.

Mason, G. & Mendl, M. (1993) Why is there no simple way of measuring animal welfare? *Animal Welfare* **2**, 301–20.

McGreevy, P.D., French, N.P. & Nicol, C.J. (1995a) The prevalence of abnormal behaviours in dressage, eventing and endurance horses in relation to stabling. *Veterinary Record* **137**, 36–7.

McGreevy, P.D., Cripps, P.J., French, N.P., Green, L.E. & Nicol, C.J. (1995b) Management factors associated with stereotypic and redirected behaviour in the Thoroughbred horse. *Equine Veterinary Journal* **2** (2), 86–91.

McGreevy, P.D. & Nicol, C.J. (1995) Behavioural and physiological consequences associated with prevention of cribbing. In: *Proceedings of the 29th International Congress of the International Society for Applied Ethology*. (eds Rutter, S.M, Rushen, J., Randle, H.D. & Eddison, J.C.). Universities Federation for Animal Welfare, Potters Bar.

Ralston, S.L. (1984) Controls of feeding in horses. *Journal of Animal Science* **59**, 1354–61.

Redbo, I., Redbo-Torstensson, P., Odberg, F.O., Hedendahl, A. & Holm, J. Factors affecting behavioural disturbances in racehorses. *Journal of Animal Science*. (In Press)

Vecchiotti, G.G. & Galanti, R. (1986) Evidence of heredity of cribbing, weaving and stall walking in Thoroughbred horses. *Livestock Production Science* **14**, 91–5.

Wiepkema, P.R. & Koolhaa, J.M. (1993) Stress and animal welfare. *Animal Welfare* **2**, 195–218.

Appendix

We hope you have enjoyed reading this book and found it useful. So that it can be improved in future editions, we would appreciate any comments that you may wish to make. These can be sent to Daniel Mills at the address below. Please note we regret but we are unable to deal with specific enquiries concerning your horse's behaviour, cases can only be examined upon referral from your veterinary surgeon.

However, if you own a horse or pony and are interested in being involved in studies about their behaviour, please copy and complete the details below and send them to Daniel Mills at the address below. Your details will then be held on a database for easy access when an appropriate study is being undertaken.

Your name:
Address:
Telephone number:

The name of your horse(s):
Type or breed:
Age:
Sex:
Use:
Size and composition of yard:
Normal housing type:
Normal diet:
Amount of exercise given each week:
Does your horse show any stereotyped behaviour patterns?
Does your horse have any other behaviour problems?
How long have you owned your horse?

I hereby give permission for the details above to be held by the De Montfort University and understand that they may be shared with individuals involved in equine research.

Signed   Date

Daniel Mills, Animal Behaviour, Welfare and Cognition Group, De Montfort University Lincoln, Caythorpe Campus, Caythorpe, Lincolnshire NG32 3EP

Index